Introduction to Primary Care Behavioral Pediatrics

This book is a comprehensive yet practical guide to the practice of primary care behavioral pediatrics for behavior analysts.

Practitioners of this subspecialty work collaboratively with caregivers, educators, pediatricians, and pediatric specialists to bring about success for primarily neurotypical children experiencing difficulties with everything from sleep and cooperation to attention, anxiety, and toileting. This book reviews the historical and theoretical foundations of the subspecialty and provides practical guidance for problem conceptualization, assessment, case formulation, treatment planning, science-based behavioral treatment, caregiver treatment adherence, multidisciplinary collaboration, and ethical practice.

A cornerstone for the field, *Introduction to Primary Care Behavioral Pediatrics* is essential for graduate students, practitioners of behavior analysis, and anyone interested in science-based pediatric behavioral healthcare.

J. Chris McGinnis, PhD, BCBA-D, is a Board Certified Behavior Analyst, licensed psychologist, and certified Health Service Psychologist based in Florida, USA. He is the CEO of McGinnis Behavioral, an outpatient behavioral health practice serving children and families, and Director of the Institute for Behavioral Pediatrics, a training and continuing education firm serving behavior analysts and other helping professionals. Dr. McGinnis has helped thousands of children and their families over more than 25 years in outpatient pediatric and clinic settings.

Introduction to Primary Care Behavioral Pediatrics

A Guide for Behavior Analysts

J. CHRIS MCGINNIS

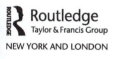
Routledge
Taylor & Francis Group

NEW YORK AND LONDON

Designed cover image: © Getty Images

First published 2024
by Routledge
605 Third Avenue, New York, NY 10158

and by Routledge
4 Park Square, Milton Park, Abingdon, Oxon, OX14 4RN

Routledge is an imprint of the Taylor & Francis Group, an informa business

© 2024 J. Chris McGinnis

ISBN: 978-1-032-44262-4 (hbk)
ISBN: 978-1-032-44243-3 (pbk)
ISBN: 978-1-003-37128-1 (ebk)

DOI: 10.4324/9781003371281

Typeset in Dante and Avenir
by MPS Limited, Dehradun

To the memory of Dr. Ron Edwards,
a card-carrying behavior analyst before there was a card to carry,
and the one to make the introduction

Contents

Acknowledgments   ix
Foreword by Patrick C. Friman, PhD, ABPP   x

Introduction   **1**

1   Definition, Niche, and Training Pathways   **11**

2   Conceptualization of the Problem   **29**

3   Assessment Methods   **46**

4   Prescriptive Behavioral Treatment and Supportive Counseling   **64**

5   Case Formulation and Treatment Planning   **80**

6   Pediatric Sleep Problems   **87**

7   Behavioral Noncompliance   **105**

8   Poor Toleration of Denial and Delay   **120**

9   Poor Self-Advocacy Skills   **124**

10   Other Clinical Problems: Anxiety, Colic, Enuresis, Encopresis, and Habits and Tics   **127**

11 **Caregiver Treatment Adherence**   **145**

12 **Multidisciplinary Collaboration**   **157**

Glossary   171
Index   184

Acknowledgments

The extraordinary influence, encouragement, and assistance of so many individuals are reflected in the very existence of this book.

I would like to express my deep gratitude to my editor, Sarah Rae, and her team at Routledge; to Pat Friman, Jon Bailey, Keith Allen, Shannon Fox-Levine, David Reitman, Luis Morales Knight, Jason Gallant, Steve Arcidiacono, Suzie Long, Pete Feuerstein, Mae Barker, Sharon Older, Sarrie Katz, Kristin Kowalczyk, Jack Scott, Jessica Holguin, Adam Holguin, Cara Shapiro, Steve Shapiro, Rina Patel, Dan Tingstrom, Joe Olmi, Bill Carlyon, Dan Daly, Amy Simpson, and Brett McCrea; and to my family, Teresa, Owen, Regan, Sue, and Kevin.

Thank you all, from the bottom of my heart.

Foreword

Patrick C. Friman, PhD, ABPP

A trained clinician, especially one with expertise in the science and practice of behavior analysis, could build a thriving behavioral pediatric practice using just this book and a few supplementary materials as guide. Had this book been available when I started my career, I would have done much more behavioral pediatric practice and much less research, the purpose of which was to create and evaluate behavioral pediatric applications, a number of which are described in this book. What I learned early remains true to this day; specifically, with deep knowledge of at least two principles of behavior (e.g., reinforcement and punishment) and workable knowledge of at least eight individual applications (e.g., see this book or Christophersen & Vanscoyoc, 2013), a clinician has the foundation for building a practice. But although that foundation is necessary, it is not sufficient. And this assertion underscores a significant virtue in this book. Specifically, in addition to describing multiple applications, it supplies guidance for collaboration with allied health professionals with a special emphasis on pediatric medical providers. Few psychology training programs include training and supervision of the professional and interpersonal skills necessary to forge a working partnership with pediatric providers. The training programs for physicians are vastly different than the training programs for most psychologists. This book heeds and addresses that potential obstacle by including sections on medical compliance and professional collaboration.

Briefly, and at the risk of some redundancy with the body of the book, I will sketch the field of behavioral pediatrics with special emphasis on its location in primary care medicine. All children in the United States have a pediatric provider. Very few children in the United States have a psychological provider at least in comparison to how many have a pediatric provider. The pediatrician is one of the most trusted professionals in the United States. The average mental health provider has to earn that kind of trust; it is rarely given automatically in the way that it's given to pediatricians. The main point here is that all children end up in pediatric medical offices multiple times over the course of their childhood but only a minority of children end up in a mental health clinic even once. Thus instead of setting up a child practice, putting up a shingle, and hoping that they will come it makes more sense to locate in an environment where they are definitely going to come. In other words, the partnership between pediatric medical providers and suitably trained behavioral providers is mutually beneficial for the providers and in turn advantageous for parents. Highly successful behavioral pediatric practices provide a virtual one-stop shop for parents who are concerned about their children's medical and behavioral needs.

In terms of establishing an effective collaboration, my view is that the behavioral pediatric provider should assume a one-down position with respect to the physician. This could be a challenge for those who insist upon parity, but parity has never been my concern. I merely want to receive referrals from pediatricians and to be invited to provide training for medical students, residents, and medical staff in general. Where I am located on the status hierarchy does not matter to me. I just want to be included. And so in a very real sense, I characterize myself as a medicine rather than a doctor and I do what I can to get pediatricians to prescribe me. Bear in mind that the pediatrician is truly trusted often to the degree that functions almost like an extended family member and thus when they recommend a mental health provider even people who are skittish about mental health are likely to comply.

Consider the scope of behavioral pediatrics: it includes 1) study of the evaluation and treatment of behavior problems in primary care settings, 2) study of the influence of biologic variables on behavior, 3) study of the effects of behavior or emotions on biologic variables, and 4) study of the interaction between biologic and behavioral factors in the evaluation, treatment, and outcome of medical problems. And as understanding of the reciprocal nature of interactions between biology and behavior and the high prevalence of behavioral concerns in pediatric settings increase, so too does the demand for behavioral pediatric services. I will discuss only one dimension of behavioral pediatric practice (albeit the largest one): routine behavior problems presenting in primary care settings. These are high-frequency, low-intensity problems that tend to be readily responsive to targeted behavioral treatments. From a colloquial perspective, these include pooping, peeing, pouting, pushing, pestering, poking, perturbing, procrastinating, picking, and puking – and a substantial number of other types of problems that don't begin with the letter P. More seriously, multiple epidemiological surveys estimate that up to 50% of all primary care pediatric visits involve, to at least some degree, behavior problems. This poses complications for the typical pediatrician for three reasons. First, their time is very limited; the average visit is only 14 minutes. That's an insufficient amount of time to fully address a home-based behavior problem effectively. Second, the average pediatrician receives very little training in the area of mental health or behavioral health. Most have only one rotation through a mental health-related service during their residency which is not enough training to establish competency for evaluation and treatment of even routine behavior problems. And third, pediatricians do not go through the rigors of medical school and residency so that they can conduct behavioral interventions such as time-out in their offices. The reason the pediatricians went into medicine is to practice medicine.

However that does not mean they are willing to surrender the care of their patients to anyone with a mental health shingle. They want practitioners who are practical, guided by science, efficient, and understand the need for detailed interdisciplinary communication at the beginning of treatment, end of treatment, and at any point that the condition becomes medically complex. As just one example of how distinct information exchange between physicians is from the exchange between psychotherapists, when physicians refer patients to other physicians the referral is always accompanied by a descriptive note, and the recipient of the referral returns correspondence pertaining to treatment progress. This kind of communication can happen between psychologists but it is the exception, not the rule. In medicine, it is the rule. And anyone interested in developing a behavioral pediatric practice would do well to observe the rule.

There are many more virtues stemming from the alliance of physicians and behavioral health providers operating in the context of behavioral pediatrics. But I need not emphasize them here because they are described very well between the covers of this book. Before I close I'd like to point out that this book has some features that are ancillary to its primary message but add to its overall quality. For example, at the end of each chapter is a précis of the contents, and at the end of the book is a detailed glossary. Frankly, the glossary itself is worth the price of admission. In closing, and to reiterate where I started, a person could go a long way toward building a successful practice by buying this book and incorporating its messages into the development of that practice. I cannot help but wish I had written it myself.

Reference

Christophersen, E. R., & Vanscoyoc, S. M. (2013). *Treatments that work with children: Empirically supported strategies for managing childhood problems* (2nd ed.). American Psychological Association.

Introduction

Several years ago I gave an invited lecture on the topic of behavioral pediatrics on the campus of the University of Central Florida. The conference was a gathering of my fellow behavior analysts, among our group the established and distinguished in the field along with students and newly certified professionals. With campy slide images of weathered treasure maps and vintage hiking compasses along for the ride, I asserted it is now time for behavior analysts to suit up for an adventurous trek deep into the wilds of pediatric behavioral healthcare.

The talk went well. All until the last few minutes of my time when a respected colleague in the back of the room raised his hand to ask a critically important question: "How do behavior analysts train for this subspecialty?" *The answer to that question isn't yet simple or clear,* I tried to explain to a room of 240 people expecting simplicity and clarity in response to a simple and clear question. Behavioral pediatrics as a subspecialty within applied behavior analysis serving the pediatric primary care population had been building steam for decades in terms of technical and procedural know-how but not much in terms of career path, particularly for behavior analysts who were not psychologists, so the path in question had remained relatively unmarked. I couldn't have been expected to have the full answer that day, but lacking a clear answer was nonetheless bothersome. It stuck with me and was my primary motivation to write this book.

See, most behavior analysts I know who practice behavioral pediatrics are psychologists. They had traveled the well-worn path toward a career in psychology and toward the end of training, as in that great Robert Frost

DOI: 10.4324/9781003371281-1

poem, happened upon a fork in the road and a path less traveled by. This was my story as well. Yet during that talk in Orlando, I was asked about the path for those who had already chosen a career in behavior analysis.

More recently I was invited by Florida State University's Jon Bailey to join the ABA Ethics Hotline as an ethicist which requires my responding to ethics-related questions pertaining to private practice and related topics. Many of these questions are from behavior analysts desiring to move into their own private practice and toward a more consultative model serving a broader clientele. To me this reflects organic momentum within the field toward serving more of the population than just one tail of the normal distribution occupied by those on the autism spectrum, but also much uncertainty given the general lack of authoritative guidance available.

That broader clientele needs us. "There is a striking shortage," say Stancin and Perrin (2014) in their article advocating collaboration between psychologists and physicians, "of qualified child mental health clinicians, especially for children younger than age 5" (p. 334). Nearly all psychologists work primarily with adults, in fact (Abramson, 2022). Over 20% of children have a behavioral health diagnosis (Merikangas *et al.*, 2010) yet historically only about 20% of *these* kids actually receive services (Centers for Disease Control and Prevention, 2022). Anxiety-based problems are most common, representing about a third (32%) of these cases, while behavioral problems are reported for 19% (Merikangas *et al.*, 2010). The demand for services has only increased since implementation of COVID-19 mitigation measures (Hill *et al.*, 2020; Leeb *et al.*, 2020; Patrick *et al.*, 2020; Samji *et al.*, 2021) and widespread adoption by children of algorithmic social media platforms which are now recognized as vectors for social contagion of behavioral health problems (Haltigan, Pringsheim, & Rajkumar, 2023; Muller-Vahl *et al.*, 2022; Olvera *et al.*, 2021). Demand far exceeds supply. There just aren't enough services available.

What about the quality of services that are available? Not good. Most forms of therapy for children unfortunately are ineffective (Jacobson, 2008; Kazdin, 2000). Despite professional associations such as the American Psychological Association and National Association of Social Workers endorsing the standard of evidence-based practice (defined as "the integration of the best available research with clinical expertise in the context of patient characteristics, culture, and preferences"; APA Presidential Task Force on Evidence-Based Practice, 2006, p. 273), approaches abound that are unsupported by science. To say nothing of the myriad scientifically unsupported approaches to childhood behavioral health problems being offered outside of the mental health field (e.g., craniosacral therapy, neurofeedback, auditory integration training; see, for example, Freeman, 2007; Cortese *et al.*, 2016; and Mudford & Cullen, 2005, respectively), nearly *half* of all licensed psychotherapists (including psychologists, social workers, and others), for example, employ New Age energy healing approaches (e.g., Thought Field Therapy and meridian tapping; Guadiano, Brown, & Miller, 2012; Guadiano *et al.*, 2015; Pignotti & Thyer, 2015). The gold standard in psychotherapy is cognitive behavioral therapy (CBT) given its evidence-based status (David, Cristea, & Hofmann, 2018); however, for two of the most common reasons children are referred for behavioral health services, attention-deficit hyperactivity disorder (ADHD) and anxiety (American Academy of Pediatrics, 2011; Merikangas *et al.*, 2010), CBT for ADHD is relatively ineffective (Knouse, 2018; Target & Fonagy, 2005) and most psychologists purporting to offer CBT for anxiety only occasionally if ever use exposure techniques, the active ingredient (44% never or rarely use them while 16% do only occasionally; Freiheit *et al.*, 2004). Assessment practices may be just as problematic; two-thirds still use the Rorschach Inkblot Test (66%; Mihura *et al.*, 2022), for example, despite its long-known problems with reliability and validity (Hunsley *et al.*, 2015; Lilienfeld, Wood, & Garb, 2000). About half of all psychologists who use the Rorschach do so with children, and 77% use it with adolescents (Mihura *et al.*, 2022).

With all this in mind, scientifically oriented readers might wonder about the extent to which psychologists and other behavioral healthcare providers are influenced by the scientific literature. Dawes (2008) estimated less than a third of all members of the American Psychological Association read scientific journals. Assuming professors and researchers make up a significant proportion of this one-third, that leaves precious few practitioners whose training led them to remain current on evidence-based approaches and methods, and on knowing how to spot, avoid, and advocate against pseudoscientific approaches and methods.

Treatment approaches and methods that are science-based do exist, however, and while research suggests clinician factors like interpersonal warmth are at least as important as the treatment itself (Norcross & Wampold, 2011), "well over five hundred scientific studies" show *"the credentials and experience of the psychotherapists are unrelated to patient outcomes"* (Dawes, 2008, p. 311, italics in the original; see also, for example, Berkovits *et al.*, 2010; Lavigne *et al.*, 2008; and Perrin *et al.*, 2014). Credentials and experience do not predict treatment effectiveness – the soundness and appropriateness of the treatment itself, along with treatment fidelity and adherence, are what matter. And despite the existence of science-based treatment approaches and methods, they are neither widely used nor widely offered to the primary care pediatric population.

All things considered, I am convinced the future of *quality primary care* pediatric behavioral healthcare can belong to behavior analysts who are already among the most science-based of all behavioral healthcare practitioners. Consistent with calls to extend the reach of behavior-analytic science (Allen, Barone, & Kuhn, 1993; Alligood & Gravina, 2021; Friman, 2006, 2010; LeBlanc, Heinicke, & Baker, 2012; Normand & Kohn, 2013; Poling, 2010), it is now time for a path to be cleared and brightly lit for behavior analysts so the quantity and quality of pediatric behavioral healthcare services may come to more closely match the burgeoning need. The main purpose of this book, therefore, is three-fold: 1) to offer guidance for behavior analysts, 2) to serve as a catalyst for growth of the subspecialty, and 3) to increase the supply of, and access to, high-quality behavioral healthcare for children and families.

Foundational Articles

As you'll notice on the coming pages, Pat Friman, a behavior analyst, psychologist, and master of his craft has been most prolific with respect to our topic; he trained under a founder of the subspecialty, Ed Christophersen, and I had the good fortune to train under Dr. Friman. Both of these individuals have been developers and supporters of the subspecialty, and three articles of theirs stand out for the purposes of this book. Keith Allen, Vincent Barone, and Brett Kuhn offered up another article well deserving of inclusion here.

The first seminal work is Christophersen's 1982 article appearing in a special issue of *Pediatric Clinics of North America* titled, "Incorporating behavioral pediatrics into primary care." He is a behavior analyst and psychologist and this was an article appearing in a medical journal with physicians as intended audience. Within the contextual backdrop of an unheeded generation-old plea by a president of the American Academy of Pediatrics (AAP) for pediatricians to address the mental health needs of children (Wilson, 1964) and finally some recent headway given efforts by the Academy to greatly expand the role of the pediatrician in the life of the child through new standards of practice, Christophersen's aim was to complement the vision with some pragmatic guidance for pediatric primary care physicians in terms of anticipatory guidance and prescriptive behavioral treatment for caregivers. This remarkable article offers protocols on toilet training, general discipline, car safety, dressing problems, mealtime problems, bedtime problems, problems in public places, and attention problems. Most pediatricians at the time desired to focus only on the medical aspects of care, and given the widely held assumption at the time that problem behavior was the result of some underlying psychiatric cause, referrals to psychiatry were made if a referral was made at all. Christophersen however insisted, "One by one, pediatricians must start learning to manage common childhood behavioral problems," and predicted,

> Over time they will not only gain confidence in their ability to do so, they will also gradually relinquish their position of underlying causes. In time, pediatrics as a field will learn to distinguish those problems that can and should be dealt with in the pediatrician's office from those that require a referral to a mental health professional.
>
> (p. 295)

A recent AAP policy statement, titled, "Mental Health Competencies for Pediatric Practice" (Foy *et al.*, 2019), reflects just how far we've come since that paper.

The second is Allen, Barone, and Kuhn's 1993 article appearing in the *Journal of Applied Behavior Analysis* titled, "A Behavioral Prescription for Promoting Applied Behavior Analysis within Pediatrics." Lamenting how behavior analysts "have developed their technology parallel to, rather than collaboratively with, pediatricians" (p. 493), therefore marginalizing themselves despite their potential for contribution, Allen and colleagues issued a roadmap for successful integration of behavior analysis with primary care pediatrics. This article mentors would-be practitioners of behavioral pediatrics with some sound practical advice: If you want to be a part of their world, you first must strive to understand it, and this may be done by joining their organizations, reading their professional journals, attending their clinic rounds and conferences, and paying attention to the kinds of problem behavior they encounter. Then, make yourself available to them: speak their language, demonstrate your effectiveness, share your behavioral technology, and communicate frequently over cases they refer to you.

The third is Friman's 2006 article appearing in the newsletter of the Association for Behavior Analysis International titled, "The Future of Applied Behavior Analysis is Under the Dome." Talking to behavior analysts, amplifying Allen and colleagues' message from over a decade prior, and reminding us of Fred Skinner's vision for the arrival of behavior analysis as a mainstream science for solving mainstream problems (see Skinner, 1953, 1987), that paper outlines Friman's vision for behavioral pediatrics as one of a number of vehicles. The past four decades have seen ABA establish itself as the treatment of choice for individuals with autism spectrum disorders, particularly for the moderate to severe end of the spectrum; while that is a significant and meaningful area of practice, this group of clients represents only a tiny percentage of the general population. The remainder is represented by the dome of the normal (or bell) curve (versus one tail of the distribution). To reach and serve this wider population, behavior analysts, Friman argues, can work in primary care medical settings as well as in homes (e.g., to reduce unintended injuries), and within the area of geriatrics.

The final, most recent work that stands out is Friman's 2010 article appearing in *The Behavior Analyst* titled, "Come on In, the Water is Fine: Achieving Mainstream Relevance through Integration with Primary Medical Care". Again, talking to behavior analysts, Friman argues, "Successfully integrating with primary care would require no new conceptual tools, no new scientific discoveries; in fact, it could be accomplished with two or three principles of behavior and a handful of applications" (p. 20). He summarizes the needs of parents of toddlers, for example, as consisting of his Ten P's: "pooping, peeing, pouting, pushing, pestering, perturbing, poking, procrastinating, picking, [and] puking" (p. 21), not to mention a few other challenges. Friman points out that while these behaviors are problematic, they are *developmentally expected and do not represent psychopathology*. Such common problems of childhood, he notes, might seem trivial but they are not trivial to the child, family, or pediatrician. There is a need here, and behavior analysts can fill it.

Dr. Friman is fond of saying that what a pediatrician writes on a prescription pad should frequently be the name of a local behavior analyst. *Be the Prescription* was, in fact, the main title of that little Orlando talk of mine. This book intends to help *you* become the prescription that pediatricians write and that parents and children need.

About This Book

In writing this book, I have attempted to provide the student as well as the practitioner of behavior analysis a comprehensive and practical guide to the practice of primary care behavioral pediatrics. What I initially conceptualized as a concise quick-start guide could have easily become a 2,000-page doorstop; in retrospect much more effort seems to have gone into culling material than in writing it. The result falls somewhere between pamphlet and tome. I outline important topics in some detail, but with plenty of references to additional sources for further study. This is not going to be the only book on your shelf, but it is a book that will help you build your professional library.

Like Friman and Christophersen, I am a psychologist and an unabashed behavior analyst. While overlap exists in this Venn diagram, the non-overlapping space is much larger in a number of important ways. Trained in both worlds and practicing a curious hybrid over nearly three decades now, my approach has largely been systematic and my focus has been the continuous improvement of treatment effectiveness, efficiency, durability, and caregiver and referral source acceptability across a broad variety of referral concerns encountered in primary care behavioral pediatrics. As Greg Hanley asserted on Matt Cicoria's excellent Behavioral Observations Podcast (in Episode #94), "If you're systematic in your approach, every case teaches something." This is absolutely true; I've seen what works and what doesn't, what's helpful and what isn't, what's efficient and what's not. The research base and my daily practice have evolved together, and the results of this evolutionary process include this book and in it its focus on behavior analysis as a toolbox for solving problems. Practitioners of all training backgrounds are hereby welcomed to consider this material en route to a greater understanding and respect for behavior analysis, its central role in behavioral pediatrics, and the daily work of its practitioners. Behavior analysts are the primary intended audience for this book, but I hope that students and practitioners of all stripes, from psychology to medicine, will find this material informative, compelling, and useful.

A final note: It has occurred to me over the course of writing this book that behavior analysts have an opportunity to spearhead a desperately needed paradigm shift in behavioral healthcare. Philosopher of science Thomas Kuhn observed that new paradigms in science tend to supplant old paradigms with which crises have arisen. A thread woven through this book is a crisis in behavioral healthcare which I argue has arisen to a large extent from a well-worn and now outdated paradigm explored in some detail in Chapter 2. "Progress in science", after all, is "progress *away from* less adequate conceptions of, and interactions with, the world" (Kuhn, 2012, p. xi, italics in the original). The movement of behavior analysts to behavioral pediatrics, and of behavioral pediatrics from science base to office-based practice, brings with it a paradigm shift, and you, dear reader, may represent the tip of the spear.

References

Abramson, A. (2022). Children's mental health is in crisis. *APA Monitor, 53,* 69.
Allen, K. D., Barone, V. J., & Kuhn, B. R. (1993). A behavioral prescription for promoting applied behavior analysis within pediatrics. *Journal of Applied Behavior Analysis, 26,* 493–502.

Alligood, C. A., & Gravina, N. E. (2021). Branching out: Finding success in new areas of practice. *Behavior Analysis in Practice, 14*, 283–289.

American Academy of Pediatrics (2011). ADHD: Clinical practice guideline for the diagnosis, evaluation, and treatment of attention-deficit/hyperactivity disorder in children and adolescents. *Pediatrics, 128*, 1007–1022.

APA Presidential Task Force on Evidence-Based Practice (2006). Evidence-based practice in psychology. *American Psychologist, 61*, 271–285.

Berkovits, M. D., O'Brien, K. A., Carter, C. G., & Eyberg, S. M. (2010). Early identification and intervention for behavior problems in primary care: A comparison of two abbreviated versions of parent-child interaction therapy. *Behavior Therapy, 41*, 375–387.

Centers for Disease Control and Prevention (2022). *Improving access to children's mental health care.* CDC. www.cdc.gov/childrensmentalhealth/access.html#ref

Christophersen, E. R. (1982). Incorporating behavioral pediatrics into primary care. *Pediatric Clinics of North America, 29*, 261–296.

Cortese, S., Ferrin, M., Brandeis, D., Holtmann, M., Aggensteiner, P., Daley, D., Santosh, P., Simonoff, E., Stevenson, J., Stringaris, A., Sonuga-Barke, E. J. S., & European ADHD Guidelines Group (2016). Neurofeedback for attention-deficit/hyperactivity disorder: Meta-analysis of clinical and neuropsychological outcomes from randomized controlled trials. *Journal of the American Academy of Child and Adolescent Psychiatry, 55*, 444–455.

David, D., Cristea, I., & Hofmann, S. G. (2018). Why cognitive behavioral therapy is the current gold standard of psychotherapy. *Frontiers in Psychiatry, 9*, 1.

Dawes, R. M. (2008). Psychotherapy: The myth of expertise. In S. O. Lilienfeld, J. Ruscio, & S. J. Lynn (Eds.), *Navigating the mindfield: A guide to separating science from pseudoscience in mental health* (pp. 311–344). Prometheus.

Foy, J. M., Green, C. M., Earls, M. F., & AAP Committee on Psychosocial Aspects of Child and Family Health, Mental Health Leadership Work Group (2019). Mental health competencies for pediatric practice. *Pediatrics, 144*(5), e20192757.

Freeman, S. K. (2007). *The complete guide to autism treatments: A parent's handbook: Make sure your child gets what works!* SKF.

Freiheit, S. R., Vye, C., Swan, R., & Cady, M. (2004). Cognitive-behavioral therapy for anxiety: Is dissemination working? *The Behavior Therapist, 27*, 25–32.

Friman, P. C. (2006). The future of applied behavior analysis is under the dome. *Association for Behavior Analysis International Newsletter, 29*(3), 4–5.

Friman, P. C. (2010). Come on in, the water is fine: Achieving mainstream relevance through integration with primary medical care. *The Behavior Analyst, 33*, 19–36.

Guadiano, B. A., Brown L. A., & Miller, I. W. (2012). Tapping their patients' problems away? Characteristics of psychotherapists using energy meridian techniques. *Research on Social Work Practice, 22*, 647–655.

Guadiano, B. A., Dalrymple, K. L., Weinstock, L. M., & Lohr, J. M. (2015). The science of psychotherapy: Developing, testing, and promoting evidence-based treatments. In S. O. Lilienfeld, S. J. Lynn, & J. M. Lohr (Eds.) (2nd ed.), *Science and pseudoscience in clinical psychology* (pp. 155–190). Guilford.

Haltigan, J. D., Pringsheim, T. M., & Rajkumar, G. (2023). Social media as an incubator of personality and behavioral psychopathology: Symptom and disorder authenticity or psychosomatic social contagion? *Comprehensive Psychiatry, 121*, 152362. 10.1016/j.comppsych.2022.152362

Hill, R. M., Rufino, K., Kurian, S., Saxena, J., Saxena, K., & Williams, L. (2020). Suicide ideation and attempts in a pediatric emergency department before and during COVID-19. *Pediatrics, 147*(3), e2020029280.

Hunsley, J., Lee, C. M., Wood, J. M., & Taylor, W. (2015). Controversial and questionable assessment techniques. In S. O. Lilienfeld, S. J. Lynn, & J. M. Lohr (Eds.) (2nd ed.), *Science and pseudoscience in clinical psychology* (pp. 42–82). Guilford.

Jacobson, N. (2008). The overselling of therapy. In S. O. Lilienfeld, J. Ruscio, & S. J. Lynn (Eds.), *Navigating the mindfield: A guide to separating science from pseudoscience in mental health* (pp. 525–538). Prometheus.

Kazdin, A. E. (2000). *Psychotherapy for children and adolescents: Direction for research and practice.* Oxford.

Knouse, L. E. (2018). Cognitive-behavioral therapies for ADHD. In R. A. Barkley (Ed.), *Attention-deficit hyperactivity disorder: A handbook for diagnosis and treatment* (4th ed., pp. 757–773). Guilford.

Kuhn, T. S. (2012). *The structure of scientific revolutions: 50th anniversary edition.* University of Chicago.

Lavigne, J. V., LeBailly, S. A., Gouze, K. R., Cicchetti, C., Pochyly, J., Arend, R., Jessup, B. W., & Binns, H. J. (2008). Treating oppositional defiant disorder in primary care: A comparison of three models. *Journal of Pediatric Psychology, 33,* 449–461.

LeBlanc, L. A., Heinicke, M. R., & Baker, J. C. (2012). Expanding the consumer base for behavior-analytic services: Meeting the needs of consumers in the 21st Century. *Behavior Analysis in Practice, 5,* 4–14.

Leeb, R. T., Bitsko, R. H., Radhakrishnan, L., Martinez, P., Njai, R., & Holland, K. M. (2020). Mental health-related emergency department visits among children aged <18 years during the COVID-19 pandemic – United States, January 1–October 17, 2020. *Morbidity and Mortality Weekly Report, 69*(45), 1675–1680.

Lilienfeld, S. O., Wood, J. M., & Garb, H. N. (2000). The scientific status of projective techniques. *Psychological Science in the Public Interest, 2,* 27–66.

Merikangas, K. R., He, J., Burstein, M., Swanson, S. A., Avenevoli, S., Cui, L., Benjet, C., Georgiades, K., & Swendsen, J. (2010). Lifetime prevalence of mental disorders in US adolescents: Results from the national comorbidity study-adolescent supplement (NCS-A). *Journal of the American Academy of Child and Adolescent Psychiatry, 49,* 980–989.

Mihura, J. L., Jowers, C. E., Dumitrascu, N., Villanueva van den Hurk, A. W., & Keddy, P. J. (2022). The specific uses of the Rorschach in clinical practice: Preliminary results from an international survey. *Rorschachiana, 43,* 25–41.

Mudford, O. C., & Cullen, C. (2005). Auditory integration training: A critical review. In J. W. Jacobson, R. M. Foxx, & J. A. Mulick (Eds.), *Controversial therapies for developmental disabilities: Fad, fashion, and science in professional practice* (pp. 351–362). Lawrence Erlbaum.

Muller-Vahl, K. R., Pisarenko, A., Jakubovski, E., & Fremer, C. (2022). Stop that! It's not Tourette's but a new type of mass sociogenic illness. *Brain, 145,* 476–480.

Norcross, J. C., & Wampold, B. E. (2011). Evidence-based therapy relationships: Research conclusions and clinical practices. *Psychotherapy, 48,* 98–102.

Normand, M. P., & Kohn, C. S. (2013). Don't wag the dog: Extending the reach of applied behavior analysis. *The Behavior Analyst, 36,* 109–122.

Olvera, C., Stebbins, G. T., Goetz, C. G., & Kompoliti, K. (2021). TikTok tics: A pandemic within a pandemic. *Movement Disorders Clinical Practice, 8,* 1163–1282.

Patrick, S. W., Henkhaus, L. E., Zickafoose, J. S., Lovell, K., Halvorson, A., Loch, S., Letterie, M., & Davis, M. M. (2020). Well-being of parents and children during the COVID-19 pandemic: A national survey. *Pediatrics*, 146(4), e2020016824.

Perrin, E. C., Sheldrick, R. C., McMenamy, J. M., Henson, B. S., & Carter, A. S. (2014). Improving parenting skills for families of young children in pediatric settings: A randomized clinical trial. *JAMA Pediatrics*, 168, 16–24.

Pignotti, M., & Thyer, B. A. (2015). New age and related novel unsupported therapies in mental health practice. In S. O. Lilienfeld, S. J. Lynn, & J. M. Lohr (Eds.) (2nd ed.), *Science and pseudoscience in clinical psychology* (pp. 191–209). Guilford.

Poling, A. (2010). Looking to the future: Will behavior analysis survive in prosper? *The Behavior Analyst*, 33, 7–17.

Samji, H., Wu, J., Ladak, A., Vossen, C., Stewart, E., Dove, N., Long, D., & Snell, G. (2021). Review: Mental health impacts of the COVID-19 pandemic on children and youth – A systematic review. *Child and Adolescent Mental Health*, doi: 10.1111/camh.12501

Skinner, B. F. (1953). *Science and human behavior*. Free Press.

Skinner, B. F. (1987). *Upon further reflection*. Century Psychology Series.

Stancin, T., & Perrin, E. C. (2014). Psychologists and pediatricians: Opportunities for collaboration in primary care. *American Psychologist*, 69, 332–343.

Target, M., & Fonagy, P. (2005). The psychological treatment of child and adolescent psychiatric disorders. In A. Roth & P. Fonagy (Eds.), *What works for whom? A critical review of psychotherapy research* (2nd ed.). Guilford.

Wilson, J. L. (1964). Growth and development of pediatrics: Presidential address–1964. *Journal of Pediatrics*, 65, 984–991.

Definition, Niche, and Training Pathways

1

Primary care behavioral pediatrics is a dynamic, emerging subspecialty and practice niche for behavior analysts serving primarily neurotypical children and their families, addressing such referral concerns as sleep and bedtime problems, behavioral noncompliance, anxiety and phobias, sibling conflict, picky eating, habits like thumbsucking, and toileting problems. Toddlerhood to late elementary school age is prime time for such services. Preadolescents and adolescents also benefit particularly with respect to sleep and anxiety-related challenges. Neurodivergent children (e.g., those with a presentation of autism spectrum disorder) are served as well, but, in contrast to the services of traditional ABA providers whose caseloads are predominantly neurodivergent, services provided by practitioners of behavioral pediatrics are on a much more time-limited basis with a relatively narrower clinical focus. Most problems encountered in behavioral pediatrics – those of high rate but low intensity – are quite common in childhood and are not diagnosable as psychopathology *per se* yet still cause suffering for the child, disrupt family life, and often get worse if not addressed early. The literature base for behavioral pediatrics has been building for over 40 years now and it is time for behavior analysts to begin putting that research into practice. At the time of this book's publication, only about 1% of the world's behavior analysts practice behavioral pediatrics (Behavior Analyst Certification Board, n.d. a), making this subspecialty one to watch over the coming years.

Behavioral pediatrics may be practiced by physicians, psychologists, or behavior analysts (Allen, Barone, & Kuhn, 1993; Friman, 2005, 2010; Friman & Blum, 2002). As asserted by two physician editors of an early textbook on

DOI: 10.4324/9781003371281-2

behavioral pediatrics, "mental health is complex and does not belong to any one group to the exclusion of others" (Greydanus & Wolraich, 1992, p. ix), and as proclaimed by a psychologist and a physician in a review paper on interdisciplinary collaboration, "blurred role boundaries between disciplines are acceptable (within the limits of professional scope of practice)" (Stancin & Perrin, 2014, p. 338). I would hasten to add *within the scope of competence* as well. The term *pediatrics*, after all, refers not only to what pediatricians do but also to the population served and to any context in which children's healthcare is provided (Friman, 2010, 2021).

Other important terminology includes primary, secondary, and tertiary care. *Primary care* refers to a clinical focus on prevention as well as amelioration of problems of low intensity that without treatment are predicted to worsen and ultimately require higher levels of care (Friman, 2006). This is relative to *secondary care* which is focused primarily on cure, and *tertiary care* which is focused on minimization of impairment from more chronic conditions.

Behavioral pediatrics is a subspecialty of clinical behavior analysis which itself represents "the application of the conceptual and methodological tools of behavior analysis to treat problems that have traditionally been characterized as mental disorders" (Behavior Analyst Certification Board, n.d. b; see also Dougher, 2000, and Hayes & Bissett, 2000). Clinical behavior analysts assess and treat such problems as anxiety, depression, substance abuse, stress, relationship problems, chronic pain, and sleep problems (Behavior Analyst Certification Board, n.d. b; Dougher, 2000; Waltz, 2010) and even delusions and hallucinations (Layng *et al.*, 2022). More narrowly, those practicing behavioral pediatrics are parenting experts with whom parents may consult and pediatricians may collaborate. They represent a type of primary care provider not for the medical aspects of care but for the social, emotional, and behavioral aspects of care. This essentially fills a gap between primary care pediatric medicine and mainstream mental health (Friman, 2010).

Behavioral pediatrics is practical in approach, prioritizing effectiveness, efficiency, durability, and acceptability of treatment. This is evident in its primary avenues of intervention which include prescriptive behavioral treatment and supportive counseling, the latter of which includes targeted health education, encouragement, and reassurance (Friman & Blum, 2002). The practitioner of behavioral pediatrics also makes referrals often in close collaboration with the child's primary care provider to ensure all needs are met.

The subspecialty is comprised of a number of domains of research and practice (Friman, 2021; Friman & Piazza, 2011), including the evaluation and treatment of common problems essentially of high rate and low intensity.

Such concerns, like bedtime refusal for example, can cause a number of downstream problems in terms of physical health (Cohen *et al.*, 2009; Hart, Cairns, & Jelalian, 2011; Walker, 2017), social and academic performance (Alfano, Ginsburg, & Kingery, 2007; Fallone, Owens, & Deane, 2002; Gruber *et al.*, 2010; Liu *et al.*, 2005; Mindell, Owens, & Carskadon, 1999), and family discord (Adams & Rickert, 1989; Alfano, Ginsburg, & Kingery, 2007; Mindell & Durand, 1993; Mindell, Kuhn, & Lewin, 2006; Mindell *et al.*, 2009). This primary care focus of behavioral pediatrics is unique in behavioral healthcare; traditional services tend to lack straightforward, efficient, and sustainable solutions for such concerns and, worse, may erroneously view such behavior as reflecting some hypothesized underlying psychiatric disorder that itself needs addressing before such referral concerns themselves may be remedied.

Other domains of research and practice in behavioral pediatrics involve the examination of the influence of physiological variables on child behavior problems, the influence of behavioral variables on child medical problems, and important contextual variables and the interaction between these, the physiological variables, and the behavioral variables. This should not be surprising given that behavior analysis, the conceptual heart of behavioral pediatrics, is at its heart contingency analysis. Pediatric toileting problems such as enuresis and encopresis represent good examples of problems involving a complex interaction between physiology, behavior, and context. Research has shown such problems to occur without an underlying psychiatric issue causing them (Friman *et al.*, 1998; Friman *et al.*, 1988) and may be efficiently and durably addressed through behavioral intervention in collaboration with the child's caregivers and pediatrician (see, for example, Christophersen & Friman, 2010).

Caregivers: Enthusiastic Cotherapists

Most primary care medical providers do not receive training in behavioral health (McMillan, Land, & Leslie, 2017) while most behavioral healthcare providers fail to offer primary care services let alone effective, science-based treatment (Addis & Krasnow, 2000; Baker, McFall, & Shoham, 2009; Dawes, 2008; Guadiano, Brown, & Miller, 2012; Jacobson, 2008; Kazdin, 2000; Lilienfeld, Lynn, & Lohr, 2008; Pignotti & Thyer, 2009; Weersing, Weisz, & Donenberg, 2002). It is therefore unsurprising that parents report inadequate access to the help they desire (Rhodes *et al.*, 2012).

The role of caregivers in their children's behavioral healthcare was essentially nonexistent until the 1960s (Roberts, 2008) and remains marginalized in traditional behavioral healthcare at least partially due to purported "confidentiality concerns" despite the fact that caregivers hold the privilege. Besides seeking effective tools, caregivers value involvement in their children's treatment and go where they are welcomed when given the choice. Until the 1960s, children had only been offered talk and play therapy largely adapted from adult psychodynamic and client-centered therapy approaches (Knopf, 1984, as cited by Reitman & McMahon, 2013). In retrospect, "therapists assumed that it was 'the child, not the therapist, who is responsible for growth and self-realization'" (p. 106). None of it worked (Levitt, 1957; Weisz & Weiss, 1993). What did work was developed in the 1960s and 1970s and involved training parents to implement procedures consistent with behavior-analytic principles (e.g., Hanf, 1970; Hanf & Kling, 1973; Patterson et al., 1975; Wahler et al., 1965). This worked because "any effective intervention strategy must assess and modify those aspects of the child's social environment that contribute to, maintain, and exacerbate problems" (Briesmeister & Schaefer, 1998, p. 8). Behavior is a product of the context in which it occurs; training caregivers fundamentally changes that context as well as empowers them, effectively immerses the child in therapy (versus 45 minutes of ineffective talk or play therapy once per week, in a context separate from that in which the problem behavior tends to occur), and promotes generalization of treatment gains. The behavioral parent training approach and literature are invaluable to practitioners of behavioral pediatrics and are covered in more detail in Chapter 4.

Pediatricians: A Most Enthusiastic Referral Source

Pediatricians are the most common primary care medical healthcare provider for children. They serve the entire population of children and see all manner of presenting concerns, treating what may be treated in the exam room and referring to specialists for all else except emergencies. Pediatricians tend to see four or more patients an hour for at least eight hours a day and, remarkably, about half of these encounters deal with behavioral, not medical, concerns (Friman, 2010; Howard, 2019; McClelland et al., 1973). The odds of referring out to psychotherapy services meeting with success, however, have been no better than a coin flip (Stein, 2008) if recommended services are received at all (Stancin & Perrin, 2014).

The most common behavioral concerns encountered in primary care pediatrics include excessive crying (otherwise known as colic) and sleep-related difficulties in infants; oppositional behavior, attention-related problems, toileting, and fears in preschool children; and academic difficulties, problem behavior at school, and peer relationship problems in school-age children (Friman, 2005). Picky eating is also a common concern of parents (Friman, 2010). Over 20% of parents of infants seek help with their children's crying. An estimated 40% of parents of toddlers desire assistance with their children's behavior and toileting, over half of all parents are seeking direction to help their children learn in school, and around 30% are looking for help with their children's sleep problems (Young et al., 1998).

The behavioral healthcare needs of children and families have only increased since COVID-19 pandemic mitigation efforts began in March of 2020 (Hill et al., 2020; Leeb et al., 2020; Patrick et al., 2020; Samji et al., 2021), with predicted long-term negative effects (Samji et al., 2021). Although many caregivers reported benefits from having increased time together during the shutdowns (Raffa et al., 2023), most agreed that the shutdowns and resulting social isolation and virtual learning were the worst things to ever happen to their child (Lurie Children's Hospital of Chicago, 2021). Worsened sleep, diet, and mental health were associated with the resulting increase in screen time (Trott et al., 2022), and over a quarter of caregivers reported a worsening of their own mental health, with disproportionate effects seen for mothers, single parents, and parents of small children (Patrick et al., 2020). Parental job loss and depression were predictive of domestic violence and child abuse seen during the shutdowns (Lawson, Piel, & Simon, 2020).

Pediatricians need assistance with children's fear and refusal around immunization and blood draw as well as with recurrent pain and general medical adherence. Challenges regarding immunization and blood draw are common; the fear of needles and diagnosable needle phobia decrease with age (Orenius et al., 2018) but fear of needles nevertheless is reported by around 65% of children ages 6 to 12 and 51% of children ages 13 to 17 (Taddio et al., 2012) while more severe needle phobia is seen in about 20% of children between the ages of 4 and 6 (Majstorovic & Veerkamp, 2003) with a mean age of onset of 5.5 years (Bienvenu & Eaton, 1998). At ages 10 and 11, the prevalence rate is 11% (Majstorovic & Veerkamp, 2003). That's a lot of kids at any age. Behavioral intervention for needle phobia involving exposure and differential reinforcement has appeared in the literature (e.g., McMurty et al., 2016; Shabani & Fisher, 2006).

Pediatric pain, seen in about 15% of children in outpatient pediatrics and particularly in obese children (Grout et al., 2018) is a leading source of pediatric healthcare utilization (Groenewald et al., 2014) and is known to impact sleep health, socialization, academics, and caregiver functioning

(Palermo, 2000; Walsh, Mulder, & Tudor, 2013). Pediatric pain has been categorized in terms of that associated with chronic disease, with observable physical injuries or traumas, with medical and dental procedures, and, most commonly, idiopathic pain, or that not associated with a well-defined or specific chronic disease or identifiable physical injury (e.g., headaches, back pain, abdominal pain; Varni, 1983). Intervention options include differential attending, biofeedback, relaxation training, contingency management, and acceptance and commitment therapy (Allen & Hine, 2015; Palermo, 2012; Pielech, Vowles, & Wicksell, 2017; see also McKeown *et al.*, 2022).

Medical adherence is another area with which pediatricians need help. Behavior analysts can fill this need, especially given that behavioral strategies are shown to be the most effective (Rapoff, 2010; Rapoff & Barnard, 1991). Chapter 11 of this book is devoted to the critically important topic of caregiver treatment adherence.

There is a lot of need in the pediatric exam room, about half of that encountered being beyond the allotted time, professional training, and reimbursement capture for most pediatricians. Collaborating with pediatricians helps them address the needs of the whole child, reduce their workload, improve outcomes, and increase satisfaction with care (Gatchel & Oordt, 2003), not to mention reduce care utilization (Finney, Riley, & Cataldo, 1991), all in turn generating more interest in and referrals to behavioral pediatrics.

Training Pathways

Most current practitioners of behavioral pediatrics found their way to the subspecialty of behavioral pediatrics via general training in psychology along with fortuitous internship and/or postdoctoral residency training. This continues to be a viable training pathway for future practitioners. A four-year undergraduate degree and another four years of graduate study followed by a one-year internship off campus and yet another year of postdoctoral residency training are typically required in order to be eligible for state licensure to practice psychology. The terminal degrees in psychology are the Doctor of Philosophy (PhD) and the Doctor of Psychology (PsyD); the former is a centuries-old degree reflecting a relative emphasis on scientific training, and the latter is a recently created degree reflecting a relative emphasis on clinical practice. Given the scientific focus of behavior analysis, a PhD is preferable.

Those already familiar with and partial to behavior analysis may find most training programs in psychology weighted with irrelevant coursework and lacking in faculty with sufficient familiarity with, or competence in, behavior analysis. Exceptions certainly exist, and in my experience these tend to be found among school psychology training programs. Psychology licensure, however, is not a requirement to practice behavioral pediatrics.

Another pathway involves entering the subspecialty via training in behavior analysis. High-quality training programs are found worldwide since the turn of the century with some offering the master's degree and some additionally offering the doctorate (PhD). The prospective student is advised to seek out a BACB-approved course sequence, preferably one with high BACB certification examination pass rates (training programs worldwide and exam pass rates may be viewed at www.bacb.com/university-pass-rates/). Once trained, the future practitioner seeks board certification in behavior analysis followed in most parts of the US by state licensure. As of this writing, 37 states have passed licensure laws (Behavior Analyst Certification Board, n.d. c).

The Behavior Analyst Certification Board (BACB), in existence since 1998 and accredited by the National Commission for Certifying Agencies (Institute for Credentialling Excellence; Carr & Nosik, 2017), offers four levels of certification: the Registered Behavior Technician (RBT), Board Certified Assistant Behavior Analyst (BCaBA), Board Certified Behavior Analyst (BCBA), and Board Certified Behavior Analyst – Doctoral (BCBA-D).

- The RBT is considered a paraprofessional-level certification, requiring a high school diploma, 40 hours of training by a BACB certificant, passing an initial competency assessment and background check, and a passing examination score. *Individuals certified at this level must be supervised.*
- The BCaBA requires an undergraduate degree with relevant coursework, supervised experience, and a passing examination score. *Individuals certified at this level must be supervised.*
- The BCBA requires a graduate degree with relevant coursework, supervised experience, and a passing examination score. *Individuals certified at this level are independent practitioners and may supervise others.*
- The BCBA-D requires a doctoral degree with relevant coursework, supervised experience, and a passing examination score. *Individuals certified at this level are independent practitioners and may supervise others.* At the time of this book's publication, the BCBA-D and the BCBA share the same criteria for certification and the *D* designation only reflects the doctoral degree.

Behavior analysts independently practicing the subspecialty of behavioral pediatrics are certified at the BCBA and BCBA-D levels and may supervise RBTs and BCaBAs within the subspecialty.

Dedicated course sequences in behavioral pediatrics offered by training programs in behavior analysis are needed. This book, as previously stated, is intended as a catalyst. Meantime, newly credentialed behavior analysts desiring a career in behavioral pediatrics are urged to seek additional and ongoing training and mentorship within the subspecialty. It is important to remember that no matter the subspecialty chosen, certification and licensure represent a minimum standard for independent practice, and the ability to meet a much higher bar should be the objective.

Practice Locations

Many options and opportunities exist for the behavior analyst practicing behavioral pediatrics in terms of practice location. I have offered services within solo and group practices as well as within exam rooms of primary care pediatric offices over the years. Some primary care practices allow rent-free use of exam rooms given the value of the services. More detailed information on colocation and integration with primary care physicians is offered in Chapter 12.

Service provision via telehealth became more technologically viable and popular with families since the COVID-19 pandemic, with research supporting its use (Neely *et al.*, 2021; Snoswell *et al.*, 2021). Services may also represent an expansion of those offered by traditional ABA therapy agencies and may be offered in the client's home under the banner of concierge or mobile services. Wherever need and unfilled niches exist, the competent behavior analyst can be welcomed and thrive, and that includes the provision of behavioral pediatric services.

Related Subspecialties

Broadly defined, behavioral pediatrics includes the medical subspecialty known as *developmental-behavioral pediatrics* representing primarily physicians' provision of medical services to children with behavioral health issues. The earliest books on our topic, *Behavioral Pediatrics: Research and Practice* (Russo & Varni, 1982) and *Clinical Behavioral Pediatrics: An Interdisciplinary Biobehavioral Approach* (Varni, 1983), were written primarily for physicians but featured behavior-analytic research as theoretical foundation (e.g., Cataldo, Russo, & Freeman, 1980; Christophersen & Gleeson, 1980). Reinforcement, response cost, and behavioral rehearsal were among those listed as "techniques of behavioral pediatrics". Furthermore,

> If the flow of talent continues to be in the movement of behaviorists *to* medicine, it is likely, therefore, that the majority of such discussion articles will focus on particular behavioral approaches. Irrespective of what logically appears to be of value, what will influence the field are data, of the highest order available, demonstrating the efficacy of behavioral techniques to produce or maintain health care behaviors. ... What is unique to behavioral approaches is their science base, a radical departure from previous psychological medicine.
>
> (Russo & Varni, 1982, p. 16; italics in the original)

The historical context of such statements is a world in which applied behaviorists were academicians; this was two decades before the BACB came into being. Although professional behavior analysts were unavailable at the time, the philosophy and methods of behavior analysis *were* available and seen as indispensable by those who had knowledge of them.

What goes by developmental-behavioral pediatrics is a subspecialty within pediatrics first recognized by the American Board of Pediatrics in 1999 (Wolraich *et al.*, 2008, p. xiii). The subspecialty's newest handbook (i.e., Augustyn & Zuckerman, 2019) offers chapters on the assessment and treatment of a dizzying array of behavioral health issues ranging from mild (e.g., breath holding) to severe (e.g., chronic medical conditions); however, a recent survey of medical practitioners of developmental-behavioral pediatrics showed a substantially narrowed focus on helping almost exclusively patients diagnosed with ADHD, autism spectrum disorder, and developmental delays (Roizen *et al.*, 2021), consistent with reports of increasing case complexity and demand within the context of increasingly fewer medical providers within the subspecialty (Bridgemohan *et al.*, 2018). Much of this work is medication management. As of this writing, there are only about 800 board-certified developmental-behavioral pediatricians, representing "an astronomical mismatch" between demand and supply and rendering developmental-behavioral pediatric services "likely the most inaccessible in all of medicine" (Godwin *et al.*, 2022). With so many children presenting with behavioral health needs within primary care settings, it stands to reason that those with milder, more common presenting concerns are falling victim to triage favoring the more severe, less common ones. That developmental-behavioral pediatrics in practice is largely abandoning children's primary care needs suggests the intended niche for developmental-behavioral pediatrics – primary care behavioral healthcare – continues to remain largely unfilled.

Pediatric psychology represents psychologists' services for children with medical conditions as well as behavioral concerns. This subspecialty within clinical child psychology was first defined in 1979 (Routh & Mesibov, 1979). Perusal of the newest handbook for that subspecialty (i.e., Roberts & Steele, 2017) finds chapters on the assessment and treatment of the behavioral dimensions of conditions such as asthma, cystic fibrosis, diabetes, cancer, traumatic brain injury, spinal cord injury, spina bifida, epilepsy, juvenile arthritis, cardiovascular disease, organ transplantation, abdominal pain-related gastrointestinal disorders, burns, and obesity. Some overlap with behavioral pediatrics and developmental-behavioral pediatrics is evidenced by other chapters on feeding problems, enuresis and encopresis, sleep, and ADHD; nonetheless, the content areas representative of the daily work of pediatric psychologists arguably are secondary and tertiary in nature, not primary.

Clinical health psychology has been defined as

> the application of knowledge and methods from all substantive fields of psychology to the promotion and maintenance of mental and physical health of the individual and to the prevention, assessment, and treatment of all forms of mental and physical disorder in which psychological influences either contribute to or can be used to relieve an individual's stress or dysfunction.
>
> (Millon, 1982, p. 9)

That's pretty broad. A more recent description put forth by the American Psychological Association (2022) proposes that it covers primary through tertiary care, "implements clinical services across diverse populations and settings to promote health and well-being and to prevent, treat and manage illness and disability", views health in general as "the confluence of psychological, social, cultural, and biological factors", and addresses such concerns as "weight management, tobacco use, pain management, psychological adjustment to serious and chronic disease, [and assesses] appropriateness for and adherence to medical treatment". Psychologists may become board certified by the American Board of Professional Psychology (ABPP) in clinical health psychology; the ABPP (n.d.) explains:

> Clinical health psychologists apply scientific knowledge of the inter-relationships among behavioral, emotional, cognitive, social, and

biological components in health and disease to the promotion and maintenance of health; the prevention, treatment, and rehabilitation of illness and disability; and the improvement of the health care system. Clinical health psychologists may be found in academic medical centers, hospitals, private practice, outpatient clinics, academia, government settings, or administration, among others.

These even broader definitions seem to cover about everything psychologists do, but with mention of pediatric behavioral healthcare provision conspicuously absent.

Pediatric and clinical health psychologists, general psychologists, child and adolescent psychiatrists, and other behavioral healthcare providers represent options for pediatricians and others for referrals. These resources are in short supply, however; only about 4% of clinical psychologists, for example, work primarily with children (Abramson, 2022). Along with the problem of supply, quality can be an issue as well, as discussed earlier. Questionable assessment techniques and treatment in behavioral healthcare for children and families unfortunately are common. Psychiatrists tend to medicalize and overpathologize common problems (Lilienfeld *et al.*, 2010) and prescribe medication that may not be necessary given less intensive and more effective treatment options available (Rosemond & Ravenel, 2008).

The niche left largely unfilled and unaddressed here is quality primary care behavioral healthcare for children and families. That's a lot of kids and a lot of demand. The push for state licensure of behavior analysts in the US over recent years has been met with some resistance on the part of psychological associations, but to the extent that resistance represents turf protection, there appears to be plenty of work for everyone, and collaboration between psychologists and behavior analysts practicing behavioral pediatrics looks to be much more synergistic than competitive.

Behavioral pediatrics – or more narrowly, *primary care behavioral pediatrics*, as contrasted with developmental-behavioral pediatrics, pediatric psychology, and related fields and subspecialties – is conceptualized as the work clinical behavior analysts and other relevant professionals do, wherever services may be delivered, in addressing the primary care behavioral healthcare needs of children via science-based assessment and treatment in collaboration with caregivers, educators, pediatricians, and other pediatric healthcare providers. The subspecialty is, in the words of

Friman and Blum (2002), a novel and perhaps even unusual approach, and one that meets the behavioral healthcare needs of children in primary care.

Key Takeaways from this Chapter

- Primary care behavioral pediatrics is a subspecialty of clinical behavior analysis serving neurotypical children and their families and addressing common behavioral problems of childhood. Behavioral pediatrics may be practiced by physicians, psychologists, or behavior analysts. Intervention avenues in behavioral pediatrics include prescriptive behavioral treatment and supportive counseling.
- The subspecialty comprises the treatment of behavior problems of high rate and low intensity, with attention to physiological variables, the influence of behavior on medical problems, and important interactions between them.
- For many years, psychotherapy with children focused on the child alone, did not involve parents, and was largely ineffective. With the advent of behavioral parent training in the 1960s, the application of behavioral principles to family interactions to in turn change child behavior showed greater effectiveness.
- Pediatricians see the entire population of children for the entire range of medical and behavioral problems, and are happy to refer out to other professionals who can solve the latter for their patients and their families. Common problems encountered by pediatricians are excessive crying (colic) and sleep-related difficulties in infants; oppositional behavior, attention-related problems, toileting, fears, and picky eating in preschool children; and academic difficulties, problem behavior at school, and peer relationship problems in school-age children. Help with needle fear and phobia, recurrent pain, and medical nonadherence is also welcomed.
- The Behavior Analyst Certification Board (BACB) offers four levels of certification: Registered Behavior Technician (RBT), Board Certified Assistant Behavior Analyst (BCaBA), Board Certified Behavior Analyst (BCBA), and Board Certified Behavior Analyst–Doctoral (BCBA-D). The BCBA and BCBA-D allow the independent practice of behavior analysis and behavioral pediatrics. Most states in the US additionally require state licensure in behavior analysis or related field (e.g., psychology) for independent practice.

- Behavior analysts practicing behavioral pediatrics may locate their services wherever there is need, from within primary care medical settings to private practice clinics and elsewhere.
- Other medical and psychological specialties in the pediatric field (e.g., developmental-behavioral pediatrics, pediatric psychology, clinical health psychology) lack a focus on primary care settings, populations, and problems.

References

Abramson, A. (2022). Children's mental health is in crisis. *APA Monitor, 53*, 69.

Adams, L. A., & Rickert, V. I. (1989). Reducing bedtime tantrums: Comparison between positive routines and graduated extinction. *Pediatrics, 84*, 756–761.

Addis, M. E., & Krasnow, A. D. (2000). A national survey of practicing psychologists' attitudes toward psychotherapy treatment manuals. *Journal of Consulting and Clinical Psychology, 68*, 331–339.

Alfano, C. A., Ginsburg, G. S., & Kingery, J. N. (2007). Sleep-related problems among children and adolescents with anxiety disorders. *Journal of the American Academy of Child and Adolescent Psychiatry, 46*, 224–232.

Allen, K. D., Barone, V. J., & Kuhn, B. R. (1993). A behavioral prescription for promoting applied behavior analysis within pediatrics. *Journal of Applied Behavior Analysis, 26*, 493–502.

Allen, K. D., & Hine, J. F. (2015). ABA applications in the prevention and treatment of medical problems. In H. S. Roane, J. E. Ringdahl, & T. S. Falcomata (Eds.), *Clinical and organizational applications of applied behavior analysis* (pp. 95–124). Academic.

American Board of Professional Psychology (n.d.). *Clinical health psychology.* ABPP. https://abpp.org/Applicant-Information/Specialty-Boards/Clinical-Health-Psychology.aspx

American Psychological Association (2022, May 16). *Clinical health psychology.* APA. www.apa.org/ed/graduate/specialize/health

Augustyn, M., & Zuckerman, B. (Eds.) (2019). *Zuckerman Parker handbook of developmental and behavioral pediatrics for primary care* (4th ed.). Wolters Kluwer.

Baker, T. B., McFall, R. M., & Shoham, V. (2009). Current status and future prospects of clinical psychology: Toward a scientifically principled approach to mental and behavioral health care. *Psychological Science in the Public Interest, 9*, 67–103.

Behavior Analyst Certification Board (n.d. a). *BACB certificant data.* www.bacb.com/BACB-certificant-data

Behavior Analyst Certification Board (n.d. b). *Clinical behavior analysis: An applied behavior analysis subspecialty.* www.bacb.com/wp-content/uploads/2020/05/Clinical-Behavior-Analysis-Fact-Sheet_190520.pdf

Behavior Analyst Certification Board (n.d. c). *U.S. licensure of behavior analysts.* Behavior Analyst Certification Board. www.bacb.com/u-s-licensure-of-behavior-analysts/

Bienvenu, O. J., & Eaton, W. W. (1998). The epidemiology of blood-injection-injury phobia. *Psychological Medicine, 28*, 1129–1136.

Bridgemohan, C., Bauer, N. S., Nielsen, B. A., DeBattista, A., Ruch-Ross, H. S., Paul, L. B., & Roizen, N. (2018). A workforce survey on developmental-behavioral pediatrics. *Pediatrics*, *141(13)*: e20172164. doi: 10.1542/peds.2017-2164

Briesmeister, J. M., & Schaefer, C. E. (Eds.) (1998). *Handbook of parent training: Parents as co-therapists for children's behavior problems* (2nd ed.). Wiley.

Carr, J. E., & Nosik, M. R. (2017). Professional credentialing of practicing behavior analysts. *Policy Insights from the Behavioral and Brain Sciences*, *4*, 3–8.

Cataldo, M. F., Russo, D. C., & Freeman, J. M. (1980). Behavior modification in a 4½ year old child with myoclonic and grand mal seizures. *Journal of Autism and Developmental Disorders*, *9*, 413–427.

Christophersen, E. R., & Friman, P. C. (2010). *Elimination disorders in children and adolescents*. Hogrefe.

Christophersen, E. R., & Gleeson, S. (1980). Research in behavioral pediatrics. *Behavior Therapist*, *3*, 13–16.

Cohen, S., Doyle, W. J., Alper, C. M., Janicki-Deverts, D., & Turner, R. B. (2009). Sleep habits and susceptibility to the common cold. *Archives of Internal Medicine*, *169*, 62–67.

Dawes, R. M. (2008). Psychotherapy: The myth of expertise. In S. O. Lilienfeld, J. Ruscio, & S. J. Lynn (Eds.), *Navigating the mindfield: A guide to separating science from pseudoscience in mental health* (pp. 311–344). Prometheus.

Dougher, M. J. (Ed.). (2000). *Clinical behavior analysis*. Context.

Fallone, G., Owens, J. A., & Deane, J. (2002). Sleepiness in children and adolescents: Clinical implications. *Sleep Medicine Reviews*, *6*, 287–306.

Finney, J. W., Riley, A. W., & Cataldo, M. F. (1991). Psychology in primary health care: Effects of brief targeted therapy on children's medical care utilization. *Journal of Pediatric Psychology*, *16*, 447–461.

Friman, P. C. (2005). Behavioral pediatrics. In M. Hersen (Ed.), *Encyclopedia of behavior modification and therapy* (Vol. 2, pp.731–739). Sage.

Friman, P. C. (2006). The future of applied behavior analysis is under the dome. *Association for Behavior Analysis International Newsletter*, *29(3)*, 4–5.

Friman, P. C. (2010). Come on in, the water is fine: Achieving mainstream relevance through integration with primary medical care. *The Behavior Analyst*, *33*, 19–36.

Friman, P. C. (2021). Behavioral pediatrics: Integrating applied behavior analysis with pediatric medicine. In W. W. Fisher, C. C. Piazza, & H. S. Roane (Eds.), *Handbook of Applied Behavior Analysis* (2nd ed., pp. 408–426). Guilford.

Friman, P. C., & Blum, N. J. (2002). Primary care behavioral pediatrics. In M. Hersen & W. Sledge (Eds.), *Encyclopedia of psychotherapy* (pp. 379–399). Academic.

Friman, P. C., Handwerk, M. L., Swearer, S. M., McGinnis, J. C., & Warzak, W. J. (1998). Do children with primary nocturnal enuresis have clinically significant behavior problems? *Archives of Pediatrics and Adolescent Medicine*, *152*, 537–539.

Friman, P. C., Mathews, J. R., Finney, J. W., Christophersen, E. R., & Leibowitz, J. M. (1988). Do encopretic children have clinically significant behavior problems? *Pediatrics*, *82*, 407–409.

Friman, P. C., & Piazza, C. C. (2011). Behavioral pediatrics: Integrating applied behavior analysis with pediatric medicine. In W. W. Fisher, C. C. Piazza, & H. S. Roane (Eds.), *Handbook of applied behavior analysis* (pp. 433–450). Guilford.

Gatchel, R. J., & Oordt, M. S. (2003). *Clinical health psychology and primary care: Practical advice and clinical guidance for successful collaboration.* American Psychological Association.

Godwin, D. L., Cervantes, J., Torres, J. Y., Ostermaier, K. K., Berry, L. N., & Voigt, R. G. (2022). A road map for academic developmental-behavioral pediatric practices to increase access. *Journal of Developmental & Behavioral Pediatrics,* doi: 10.1097/DBP.0000000000001132

Greydanus, D. E., & Wolraich, M. L. (1992). *Behavioral pediatrics.* Springer-Verlag.

Groenewald, C. B., Essner, B. S., Wright, D., Fesinmeyer, M. D., & Palermo, T. M. (2014). The economic costs of chronic pain among a cohort of treatment-seeking adolescents in the United States. *Journal of Pain, 15,* 925–933.

Grout, R. W., Thompson-Fleming, R., Carroll, A. E., & Downs, S. M. (2018). Prevalence of pain reports in pediatric primary care and association with demographics, body mass index, and exam findings: A cross-sectional study. *BMC Pediatrics, 18,* 363. 10.1186/s12887-018-1335-0

Gruber, R., Laviolette, R., Deluca, P., Monson, E., Cornish, K., & Carrier, J. (2010). Short sleep duration is associated with poor performance on IQ measures in healthy school-age children. *Sleep Medicine, 11,* 289–294.

Guadiano, B. A., Brown L. A., & Miller, I. W. (2012). Tapping their patients' problems away? Characteristics of psychotherapists using energy meridian techniques. *Research on Social Work Practice, 22,* 647–655.

Hanf, C. (1970). *Shaping mothers to shape their children's behavior.* Unpublished manuscript, University of Oregon Medical School.

Hanf, C., & Kling, J. (1973). *Facilitating parent-child interaction: A two-stage training model.* Unpublished manuscript, University of Oregon Medical School.

Hart, C. N., Cairns, A., & Jelalian, E. (2011). Sleep and obesity in children and adolescents. *Pediatric Clinics of North America, 58,* 715–733.

Hayes, S. C., & Bissett, R. T. (2000). Behavioral psychotherapy in the rise of clinical behavior analysis. In J. Austin & J. E. Carr (Eds.), *Handbook of applied behavior analysis* (pp. 231–245). Context.

Hill, R. M., Rufino, K., Kurian, S., Saxena, J., Saxena, K., & Williams, L. (2020). Suicide ideation and attempts in a pediatric emergency department before and during COVID-19. *Pediatrics, 147(3),* e2020029280.

Howard, B. J. (2019). Managing behavior in primary care. In M. Augustyn and B. Zuckerman (Eds.), *Zuckerman Parker handbook of developmental and behavioral pediatrics for primary care* (4th ed.) (pp. 73–78). Wolters Kluwer.

Jacobson, N. (2008). The overselling of therapy. In S. O. Lilienfeld, J. Ruscio, & S. J. Lynn (Eds.), *Navigating the mindfield: A guide to separating science from pseudoscience in mental health* (pp. 525–538). Prometheus.

Kazdin, A. E. (2000). *Psychotherapy for children and adolescents: Direction for research and practice.* Oxford.

Knopf, I. J. (1984). *Childhood psychopathology: A developmental approach.* Prentice Hall.

Lawson, M., Piel, M. H., & Simon, M. (2020). Child maltreatment during the COVID-19 pandemic: Consequences of parental job loss on psychological and physical abuse towards children. *Child Abuse and Neglect, 110 (Part 2),* doi: 10.1016/j.chiabu.2020.104709

Layng, T. V. J., Andronis, P. T., Codd III, R. T., & Abdel-Jalil, A. (2022). *Nonlinear contingency analysis: Going beyond cognition and behavior in clinical practice.* Routledge.

Leeb, R. T., Bitsko, R. H., Radhakrishnan, L., Martinez, P., Njai, R., & Holland, K. M. (2020). Mental health-related emergency department visits among children aged <18 years during the COVID-19 pandemic – United States, January 1–October 17, 2020. *Morbidity and Mortality Weekly Report, 69(45),* 1675–1680.

Levitt, E. E. (1957). Results of psychotherapy with children: An evaluation. *Journal of Consulting Psychology, 21,* 189–196.

Lilienfeld, S. O., Lynn, S. J., & Lohr, J. M. (2008). Science and pseudoscience in clinical psychology: Initial thoughts, reflections, and considerations. In S. O. Lilienfeld, J. Ruscio, & S. J. Lynn (Eds.), *Navigating the mindfield: A guide to separating science from pseudoscience in mental health* (pp. 57–74). Prometheus.

Lilienfeld, S. O., Lynn, S. J., Ruscio, J., & Beyerstein, B. L. (2010). *50 great myths of popular psychology: Shattering widespread misconceptions about human behavior.* Wiley-Blackwell.

Liu, X., Liu, L., Owens, J. A., & Kaplan, D. L. (2005). Sleep patterns and sleep problems among school children in the United States and China. *Pediatrics, 115,* 241–249.

Lurie Children's Hospital of Chicago (2021). *Children's mental health during the COVID-19 pandemic.* www.luriechildrens.org/en/blog/childrens-mental-health-pandemic-statistics/

Majstorovic, M., & Veerkamp, J. S. (2003). Relationship between needle phobia and dental anxiety. *Journal of Dentistry for Children (Chicago, IL), 71,* 201–205.

McClelland, C. Q., Staples, W. I., Weisberg, I., & Bergen, M. E. (1973). The practitioner's role in behavioral pediatrics. *The Journal of Pediatrics, 82,* 325–331.

McKeown, C. A., Vollmer, T. R., Cameron, M. J., Kinsella, L., & Shaibani, S. (2022). Pediatric pain and neurodevelopmental disorders: Implications for research and practice in behavior analysis. *Perspectives on Behavior Science, 45,* 597–617.

McMillan, J. A., Land, M., & Leslie, L. K. (2017). Pediatric residency education and the behavioral and mental health crisis: A call to action. *Pediatrics, 139(1),* e20162141. 10.1542/peds.2016-2141

McMurty, C. M., Taddio, A., Noel, M., Antony, M. M., Chambers, C. T., Asmundson, G. J. G., Riddell, R. P., Shah, V., MacDonald, N. E., Rogers, J., Bucci, L. M., Mousmanis, P., Lang, E., Halperin, S., Bowles, S., Halpert, C., Ipp, M., Rieder, M. J., Robson, K., Uleryk, E., Bleeker, E. V., Dubey, V., Hanrahan, A., Lockett, D., & Scott, J. (2016). Exposure-based interventions for the management of individuals with high levels of needle fear across the lifespan: A clinical practice guideline and call for further research. *Cognitive Behaviour Therapy, 45(3),* 217–235, 10.1080/16506073.2016.1157204

Millon, T. (1982). On the nature of clinical health psychology. In T. Millon, C. J. Green, & R. B. Meagher (Eds.), *Handbook of clinical health psychology* (pp. 1–27). Plenum.

Mindell, J. A., & Durand, V. M. (1993). Treatment of childhood sleep disorders: Generalization across disorders and effects on family members. *Journal of Pediatric Psychology, 18,* 731–750.

Mindell, J. A., Kuhn, B. R., & Lewin, D. S. (2006). Behavioral treatment of bedtime problems and night wakings in infants and young children. *Sleep, 29,* 1263–1276.

Mindell, J. A., Owens, J. A., & Carskadon, M. A. (1999). Developmental features of sleep. *Child and Adolescent Psychiatric Clinics of North America, 8,* 695–725.

Mindell, J. A., Telofski, L., Weigand, B., & Kurtz, E. S. (2009). A nightly bedtime routine: Impact on sleep in young children and maternal mood. *Sleep, 32,* 599–606.

Neely, L., MacNaul, H., Gregori, E., & Cantrell, K. (2021). Effects of telehealth-mediated behavioral assessments and interventions on client outcomes: A quality review. *Journal of Applied Behavior Analysis, 54,* 484–510.

Orenius, T., Saila, H., Mikola, K., & Ristolainen, L. (2018). Fear of injections and needle phobia among children and adolescents: An overview of psychological, behavioral, and contextual factors. *Sage Open Nursing, 4*, 1–8. DOI 10.1177/2377960818759442

Palermo, T. M. (2000). Impact of recurrent and chronic pain on child and family daily functioning: A critical review of the literature. *Journal of Developmental and Behavioral Pediatrics, 21*, 58–69.

Palermo, T. M. (2012). *Cognitive-behavioral therapy for chronic pain and children and adolescents*. Oxford University.

Patrick, S. W., Henkhaus, L. E., Zickafoose, J. S., Lovell, K., Halvorson, A., Loch, S., Letterie, M., & Davis, M. M. (2020). Well-being of parents and children during the COVID-19 pandemic: A national survey. *Pediatrics, 146*(4), e2020016824.

Patterson, G. R., Reid, J. B., Jones, R. R., & Conger, R. E. (1975). *A social learning approach to family intervention: Families with aggressive children* (Vol. 1). Castalia.

Pielech, M., Vowles, K. E., & Wicksell, R. (2017). Acceptance and Commitment Therapy for pediatric chronic pain: Theory and application. *Children, 4*, doi 10.3390/children4020010

Pignotti, M. G., & Thyer, B. A. (2009). Some comments on energy psychology: A review of the evidence: Premature conclusions based on incomplete evidence? *Psychotherapy, 46*, 257–261.

Raffa, B. J., Heerman, W. J., Lampkin, J., Perrin, E. M., Flower, K. B., Delamater, A. M., Yin, H. S., Rothman, R. L., Sanders, L., & Schilling, S. (2023). Parental perspectives on the impact of the COVID-19 pandemic on infant, child, and adolescent development. *Journal of Developmental and Behavioral Pediatrics*, doi: 10.1097/DBP.0000000000001166

Rapoff, M. A. (2010). *Adherence to pediatric medical regimens* (2nd ed.). Springer.

Rapoff, M. A., & Barnard, M. U. (1991). Compliance with pediatric medical regimens. In J. A. Kramer & B. Spilker (Eds.), *Patient compliance in medical practice and clinical trials* (pp. 73–98). Raven.

Reitman, D., & McMahon, R. J. (2013). Constance "Connie" Hanf (1917–2002): The mentor and the model. *Cognitive and Behavioral Practice, 20*, 106–116.

Rhodes, A., Sciberras, E., Oberklaid, F., South, M., Davies, S., & Efron, D. (2012). Unmet developmental, behavioral, and psychosocial needs in children attending pediatric outpatient clinics. *Journal of Developmental and Behavioral Pediatrics, 33*, 469–478.

Roberts, M. W. (2008). Parent training. In M. Hersen & A. M. Gross (Eds.), *Handbook of clinical psychology* (Vol. 2; pp. 653–693). Wiley.

Roberts, M. C., & Steele, R. G. (Eds.) (2017). *Handbook of pediatric psychology* (5th ed). Guildford.

Roizen, N. J., Ruch-Ross, H. S., Bauer, N. S., Nielsen, B. A., DeBattista, A., Paul, L. B., & Bridgemohan, C. (2021). Developmental-behavioral pediatrics 13 years after the first board certification: Evolving subspecialty. *Journal of Developmental and Behavioral Pediatrics, 42*, 83–90.

Rosemond, J., & Ravenel, B. (2008). *The diseasing of America's children: Exposing the ADHD fiasco and empowering parents to take back control*. Thomas Nelson.

Routh, D. K., & Mesibov, G. B. (1979). The editorial policy of the Journal of Pediatric Psychology. *Journal of Pediatric Psychology, 4*, 1–3.

Russo, D. C., & Varni, J. W. (1982). Behavioral pediatrics. In D. C. Russo & J. W. Varni (Eds.) *Behavioral pediatrics: Research and practice* (pp. 3–24). Plenum.

Samji, H., Wu, J., Ladak, A., Vossen, C., Stewart, E., Dove, N., Long, D., & Snell, G. (2021). Review: Mental health impacts of the COVID-19 pandemic on children and youth – A systematic review. *Child and Adolescent Mental Health*, doi: 10.1111/camh.12501

Shabani, D. B. & Fisher, W. W. (2006). Stimulus fading and differential reinforcement for the treatment of needle phobia in a youth with autism. *Journal of Applied Behavior Analysis, 39,* 449–452.

Snoswell, C. L., Chelberg, G., DeGuzman, K. R., Haydon, H. H., Thomas, E. E., Caffrey, L. J., & Smith, A. C. (2021). The clinical effectiveness of telehealth: A systematic review of meta-analyses from 2010 to 2019. *Journal of Telemedicine and Telecare*, 10.1177/1357633X211022907

Stancin, T., & Perrin, E. C. (2014). Psychologists and pediatricians: Opportunities for collaboration in primary care. *American Psychologist, 69,* 332–343.

Stein, M. T. (2008). Strategies to enhance developmental and behavioral services in primary care. In M. L. Wolraich, D. D. Drotar, P. H. Dworkin, & E. C. Perrin (Eds.), *Developmental-behavioral pediatrics* (pp. 887–903). Mosby.

Taddio, A., Ipp, M., Thivakaran, S., Jamal, A., Parikh, C., Smart, S., & Katz, J. (2012). Survey of the prevalence of immunization non-compliance due to needle fears in children and adults. *Vaccine, 30,* 4807–4812.

Trott, M., Driscoll, R., Iraldo, E., & Pardhan, S. (2022). Changes and correlates of screen time in adults and children during the COVID-19 pandemic: A systematic review and meta-analysis. *eClinicalMedicine, 48,* 101452. 10.1016/j.eclinm.2022.101452

Varni, J. W. (1983). *Clinical behavioral pediatrics: An interdisciplinary biobehavioral approach*. Pergamon.

Wahler, R. G., Winkel, G. H., Peterson, R. F., & Morrison, D. C. (1965). Mothers as behavior therapists for their own children. *Behavior Research and Therapy, 3,* 113–124.

Walker, M. (2017). *Why we sleep: Unlocking the power of sleep and dreams*. Scribner.

Walsh, C. E., Mulder, E., & Tudor, M. E. (2013). Predictors of parent stress in a sample of children with ASD: Pain, problem behavior, and parental coping. *Research in Autism Spectrum Disorders, 7,* 256–264.

Waltz, T. (2010). Clinical behavior analysis. *Inside Behavior Analysis, 2,* http://www.abainternational.org/ABA/newsletter/IBAvol2iss2/SIGs/clinicalSIG.asp.

Weersing, V. R., Weisz, J. R., & Donenberg, G. R. (2002). Development of the Therapy Procedures Checklist: A therapist-report measure of technique use in child and adolescent treatment. *Journal of Clinical Child Psychology, 31,* 168–180.

Weisz, J. R., & Weiss, B. (1993). *Effects of psychotherapy with children and adolescents*. Sage.

Wolraich, M. L., Drotar, D. D., Dworkin, P. H., & Perrin, E. C. (Eds.) (2008). *Developmental-behavioral pediatrics: Evidence and practice*. Mosby.

Young, K. T., Davis, K., Schoen, C., & Parker, S. (1998). Listening to parents: A national survey of parents with young children. *Archives of Pediatrics and Adolescent Medicine, 152,* 255–262.

Conceptualization of the Problem 2

Conceptualization matters. Treatments are chosen based on how problems are conceptualized (Evans, 2005). There are lots of theories and models, some science-based and some less so, in behavioral healthcare. Most, it would appear, have been developed for secondary and tertiary care clients, and our current healthcare system (along with its reimbursement contingencies) has evolved with these models and clients in mind. Primary care behavioral pediatrics, on the other hand, is rather unique across the behavioral healthcare landscape in that its focus is more on prevention and amelioration of low-intensity problems before they worsen. It is also focused on child clients in the context of family life, not on individuals considered in isolation. This pediatric primary care focus, along with a commitment to science-based practice, tend to result in its practitioners having a very different take on presenting problems.

The Biomedical Model of Mental Illness

The dominant model at the moment for understanding problem behavior is the biomedical model, which involves the concept of mental disorders that are considered medical disease states caused by faulty genes, brain structure, or brain function (Abramowitz, 2015; Edelbrock & Costello, 1984). Underlying this model is the philosophy of mentalism (a term with both positive and pejorative connotation; Burgos & Killeen, 2019) reflecting an assumption of an inner metaphysical dimension, such as the mind, that causes behavior (Cooper,

DOI: 10.4324/9781003371281-3

Heron, & Heward, 2020; Johnston, Pennypacker, & Green, 2020; Moore, 2003). This metaphysical inner dimension is accessed through the use of hypothetical constructs which are speculative concepts created to account for what is observed (Moore, 1995; Shermer, 2002; note that hypothetical constructs should not be confused with *analytic* constructs which represent intervening variables capable of being tested empirically, e.g., positive reinforcement; see MacCorquodale & Meehl, 1948, and Lovasz & Slaney, 2013, for discussion). The mental disorders diagnosed by healthcare professionals are hypothetical constructs, and those formally recognized at any given moment are cataloged in the *Diagnostic and Statistical Manual of Mental Disorders* (DSM, now in a "text revision" of its fifth edition; American Psychiatric Association, 2022; see also those pertaining to behavioral health found in the World Health Organization's 2019 *International Classification of Diseases*, or ICD).

Problems with the Biomedical Model

Despite the longstanding common usage of the biomedical model, it has not been very successful from a scientific standpoint (Hayes, Sanford, & Feeney, 2015). The mental disorders in use are neither adequately reliable nor biologically valid and decades of well-funded biomedical research have yet to identify a single biological variable useful in diagnosis (Deacon & McKay, 2015). That is, no medical test exists to objectively verify the existence of any such conditions in individual clients or in general. Although page 29 of the DSM-5-TR cautions "a diagnosis does not carry any necessary implications regarding the etiology or causes of the individual's mental disorder", certain problem behavior in childhood is referred to as "neurodevelopmental" in nature on the very next page. A few pages later, "differences in brain processes that produce impairments" are mentioned (p. 35).

The phenomenon of the chemical imbalance is taken for granted by many professionals and the general public and yet normative measurement ranges for neurotransmitters have never been established (Lacasse & Leo, 2005; see also Kirsch, 2010, and Lacasse & Leo, 2015). The class of antidepressant medications known as selective serotonin reuptake inhibitors, or SSRIs, for example, has been in widespread use for decades yet upon close inspection these medications appear no better for depression than placebo (Moncrieff *et al.*, 2022; see also Kirsch *et al.*, 2002) and to worsen long-term outcome (Whitaker, 2015). A recent paper closely examining fluoxetine (brand name: Prozac) trial data concluded this SSRI to be ineffective and unsafe for use with children and adolescents presenting with depression

(Gotzsche & Healy, 2022). The "serotonin hypothesis" upon which the manufacture of these medications is based, after all, remains but an unsupported hypothesis (Ang, Horowitz, & Moncrieff, 2022).

The practice of diagnosing hypothetical constructs and not verifiable disease states inherently involves some logical error. This may be illustrated by taking a typical conversation between caregiver and professional with respect to, for example, ADHD, the most commonly diagnosed mental disorder of childhood (American Academy of Pediatrics, 2011) and one with which 10 percent of all children in the US are diagnosed (Centers for Disease Control and Prevention, 2022).

> The caregiver asks, "Why is my child so inattentive, hyperactive, and impulsive?" to which the professional confidently replies after some assessment, "Because he has ADHD."

The professional here is *reifying* a hypothetical construct, talking about a concept as if it were an actual, biologically verifiable disease state. The reply is also *reductionist* in nature; surely there are more causal factors to consider (more on this later).

Psychologist Robert Woodworth cautioned in his 1929 psychology textbook, "Instead of memory, we should say remembering; instead of thought, we should say thinking; instead of sensation we should say seeing, hearing, etc. But, like other learned branches, psychology is prone to transform its verbs into nouns." He continued, "Then what happens? We forget that our nouns are merely substitutes for verbs, and go hunting for the *things* denoted by the nouns; but there are no such things, there are only the activities that we started with: seeing, remembering, and so on" (pp. 5–6; italics in the original and punctuation modernized). We have continued to make this mistake for a century.

> The caregiver then asks the professional, "How do you really know he has ADHD?" to which the professional replies, "Because of his inattention, hyperactivity, and impulsivity, as I have evaluated. This is how everyone does it."

The professional is now engaging in *circular logic*, using the conclusion to validate the premise. There are also the fallacies of *argumentum ab auctoritate* and *argumentum ad populum*, that something must be true because experts say so and because everybody does it this way, respectively. We might also consider the *fundamental attribution error* in the professional's diagnosis of the problem; this error refers to the general tendency to blame something neurological or characterological in others for their problem behavior or misfortunes while more charitably blaming circumstances for our own (Friman, 2021).

Neuroscience and Problem Behavior

Research involving brain imaging has compared those diagnosed with various mental disorders with those not diagnosed and has found differences in brain structure and function. To continue with the example of ADHD, multiple lines of research appear to implicate structural brain abnormalities (e.g., relatively smaller prefrontal-striatal regions and underdeveloped white matter integrity; Castellanos *et al.*, 1996; and van Ewijk *et al.*, 2012, respectively) and functional brain abnormalities (e.g., relatively less blood flow to the right prefrontal cortex; Barkley, 2018). Research has also suggested ADHD is highly heritable (Nikolas & Burt, 2010). Yet such research implicating these ostensibly causal factors is correlational in nature, telling us differences exist but not *why* they exist or whether those differences reliably result in different behavioral topographies.

Fascinatingly, other lines of research suggest that the brain, and gene expression, are altered by experience. The human brain comprises more than a trillion neurons, involving up to a quadrillion connections among them (Ehrlich, 2000), rewiring itself constantly in response to behavior and context. This highly dynamic process involving molecular, cellular, structural, and physiological events (Kleim & Jones, 2008) is known as neuroplasticity (*plastic* means malleable). The brain is altered at least briefly by virtually every experience, with more lasting neurological changes occurring when the experience is more frequent, relevant, or intense (Kolb & Gibb, 2008). And as described by Burton (2013), "We learn through trial and error. So does our brain; it creates a number of connections in an attempt to solve a problem. Once the optimal solution is achieved, the other, less useful connections are no longer necessary and are winnowed away" (p. 185). The strengthening of these connections is referred to as long-term potentiation, which serves to lock in fragile new skills as they evolve into habit patterns.

Neuroplasticity itself is mediated by epigenetic influences. The human genome is comprised of some 30,000 genes affecting approximately 100 trillion cells (Molfese, 2011). Expression of those genes, or phenotype, is altered by life experience via DNA methylation and histone acetylation among other mechanisms, without altering the DNA sequence, or genotype. This process provides the individual, from an evolutionary perspective, a mechanism for instant adaptation to the environment (Mychasiuk, 2015). As explained by Simons and Klopack (2015), "In contrast to the old view of the deterministic gene, the new paradigm places the environment center stage" (p. 575), with neuroplastic and epigenetic alterations producing what amounts to a record of the experiences of the individual (Molfese, 2011).

Consider how children learn – or fail to learn – academic skills. We know academic instruction can be effective or ineffective depending on whether there are clear objectives from the start, stepwise introduction of prerequisite skills, models of competent and accurate responding, opportunities for accurate responding, and immediate congratulatory or corrective feedback given (Fredrick & Hummel, 2004). A teaching approach known as Direct Instruction, for example, follows these principles and its effectiveness is far superior to other educational approaches (see National Institute for Direct Instruction, n.d., and the Project Follow Through study). Children who are not educated using such evidence-based instructional methods are more likely to fall behind academically. The clinical problem – being behind academically – is thereafter conceptualized *not* as resulting from inadequate instruction, but instead from something neurologically or genetically awry: a learning disability.

Only eight weeks of demonstrably effective remedial instruction, however, renders the brains of children diagnosed with dyslexia (or reading disability; Simos *et al.*, 2002) and dyscalculia (or math disability; Iuculano *et al.*, 2015) functionally indistinguishable from those of children without learning disability diagnoses upon imaging. Differences in neurological function were seen at baseline, however. Academic instruction, whether effective or ineffective, changes the brain.

Here is more evidence of experience changing the brain. A demonstrably effective nine-week course of therapy for social anxiety was shown to reduce gray matter volume and neural responsivity of the amygdala, a critical part of the "fear circuit" of the brain (Mansson *et al.*, 2016). Meditation has been shown to not only affect gray matter but also white matter, or the interconnections between gray matter regions (National Institutes of Health, 2013). Intensive practice of specific skills appears to increase gray matter volume in relevant brain regions for pianists (Gaser & Schlaug, 2003) and taxi drivers (Woollett & Maguire, 2011). Operant conditioning is known to engage structural and functional neuroplasticity from the level of single neuron all the way up to large neural networks (Schlinger, 2015).

Astonishingly, we also know that simply mentally rehearsing a task induces neuroplastic changes (Kays, Hurley, & Taber, 2012). Engaging neuroplasticity is the whole point of rehabilitation following a stroke in order to achieve functional recovery (Bowden, Woodbury, & Duncan, 2013). And, perhaps most compelling is the fact that identical twins do not have identical brains (Kates et al., 1998) because they are living different lives.

Hayes and colleagues (2015) may have said it best when it comes to the relationship between brain and behavior:

> Cast as a physical object, a gene is just a sequence of nucleotides; the brain is just a neurobiological organ. Cast as part of an evolving system, a gene (or the brain) alters the functioning of other biological processes and evolved because it does so; a gene (or the brain) impacts learning, cognition, and culture and it is in turn impacted by these same processes; a given gene may be up and down regulated by myriad biological processes such as methylation, or the folding of DNA into proximal loops, and these regulatory processes are themselves regulated by environment and behavior. The brain or genes become dependent variables just as much as independent ones. This means it is impossible to separate out biological elements from the systems in which they are embedded over time – they need to be understood historically and in context. ... Any statement that genes or the brain cause psychopathology misses the ongoing evolutionary and systemic complexity of the obtained relationships once even a short time frame is added to the picture.
>
> (p. 224)

An Alternative Model

Our longstanding fealty to the biomedical model and its underlying philosophy of mentalism has regrettably consigned much of modern behavioral health research and practice to the status of soft, or special, science (Rosenberg & McIntyre, 2020; see also Scull, 2021, and Uher & Rutter, 2012). At the very least, science requires the use of falsifiable concepts (Popper, 1959); yet the hypothetical construct, lying at the center of modern behavioral healthcare, is by its very nature unfalsifiable.

An alternative philosophy to mentalism, however, is that of functionalism, from which sprung "the most powerful idea ever invented by mankind for understanding, knowing, and approaching human behavior"

(Friman, 2017, p. 176): that behavior occurs not due to some internal cause but as a function of present and historical circumstances. Psychologist B. F. Skinner (1938, 1953) led this charge, replacing the hypothetical construct with the *operant*, or act-in-context, as unit of analysis. This philosophical revolution allowed behavior analysis to become the preeminent vehicle for the establishment of a hard, or natural, science of behavior (Baum, 2018; Fisher, Groff, & Roane, 2011; Fraley & Vargas, 1986; Glenn, Ellis, & Greenspoon, 1992; Johnston, Pennypacker, & Green, 2020).

This move to a functionalist approach also rendered psychopathological interpretations of problem behavior obsolete even if they remain in common use. Behavior-analytic conceptualization of problem behavior focuses not on behavioral topography (i.e., what it looks like) but on behavioral function; behavior-analytic assessments focus on the ascertainment of which skills to teach to whom and what changes to the social and physical environment need to be made in order to achieve a desired outcome. Behavior analysts therefore are engineers, applying science-based principles to real-world problems in order to change future probabilities of certain behaviors and outcomes.

Returning again to the example of ADHD: The question, "Does ADHD exist?" is perhaps most accurately answered,

> *Yes, the hypothetical construct of ADHD exists, but "ADHD" is not the cause of the behavior used to diagnose it.*

This may be followed up with

> *No one has ADHD although their behavior may satisfy diagnostic criteria for it.*

This is also the case for any other DSM diagnosis. Additionally, the question, "If 'ADHD' is not the cause of its symptoms, then what is?" might be answered with

> *I'm certain there are many factors, some of which we may be able to identify and influence, and in turn get to a point at which your child's behavior no longer satisfies criteria for it.*

A sufficiently complete understanding of behavior, after all, is demonstrated in our ability to predict and influence it (Schlinger, 1995), and this is most effectively done by engaging lawful relationships between behavior and context; hypothetical constructs, on the other hand, merely describe, but do not explain, the phenomena to which they refer. It may be useful to remember that hypothetical constructs essentially represent verbal behavior (i.e., a story about events) and are themselves a function of historical and present circumstances.

It appears likely that to whatever extent genetics, brain structure, or brain function play a role in problem behavior, it is downstream from the contextual practice of the behavior. That is, enduring patterns of problem behavior are most likely the result of habit patterns developed from repetitive practice within particular situational contexts, triggered by those situational contexts, and made more likely to be triggered by those situational contexts by epigenetic and neuroplastic processes. In terms of treatment, this means that epigenetic and neuroplastic processes may be engaged to the child's benefit via the teaching of replacement behaviors and engineering the social and physical environment to trigger only those replacement behaviors. Altering skill repertoire and environment alters behavior, which in turn alters the brain, which then in turn improves maintenance of the new repertoire. Perhaps Aristotle said this much more succinctly over two millennia ago: *We are what we repeatedly do; excellence, then, is not an act but a habit.*

The relationship between functionalist approaches to problem behavior and our cultural penchant for mentalistic diagnosis may sometimes be an uneasy one but they can, however, and must coexist for now, given the value of multidisciplinary collaboration and extant contingencies of funding for services and research. Behavior analysts, finding behavior lawful regardless of diagnosis (Dinsmoor, 1992), might choose to view diagnosis simply as verbal shorthand for topographical classes of behavior. Behavior analysis is extradiagnostic in nature, fully capable of operating outside of topographical diagnostic classification systems; yet, it is also transdiagnostic given its broad applicability across diagnoses. Moreover, according to Baer, Wolf, and Risley (1987), diagnosis "represents some behavioral reality not yet analyzed as such," and such constructs "might well be analyzed behavior analytically, perhaps with great profit to us and those disciplines, and thus to our roles within those disciplines" (p. 315). This in fact represents the origin story of behavioral pediatrics some 40 years ago (e.g., Christophersen, 1982). The DSM is authored and published by an association of psychiatrists but is used by all manner of behavioral health professionals including psychologists, clinical social workers, and other mental health therapists. It may be a tool for the behavior analyst as well. Access to services may be increased via its use, and those preparing for entrance into the subspecialty who seek and receive appropriate training and supervision in DSM diagnosis will likely hold a competitive advantage in some practice settings over those who do not. The behavior analyst who consults the DSM is ultimately responsible for ensuring topographical diagnosis is within his or her scope of practice and competence.

Other Critical Considerations for Problem Conceptualization

Friman and Blum (2002), in describing the theoretical bases underlying behavioral pediatrics, offered helpful ways of conceptualizing problem behavior typically encountered in practice. Among these are consideration of individual differences and temperament, how everyday language affects behavior for better or worse, the role of behavioral practice (versus simply talking about behavior), and how learning is largely governed by repetition of contrasting consequences for specific behaviors. A review of this important guidance is offered below.

Temperament and Individual Differences

The concepts of temperament and individual differences have long been revered in behavioral healthcare at least in an academic sense (see, for example, Thomas & Chess, 1977), yet potential mismatch between those individual differences and the demands and other characteristics of the environment does not appear to be much of a consideration in traditional practice. Consideration of this potential mismatch nonetheless is critical in the effective conceptualization of problem behavior. The child's conceptual, verbal, and physical capabilities may be overestimated by caregivers, in turn occasioning an increasingly coercive pattern of interaction. Moreover, as explained by Friman and Blum, the cluster of temperamental characteristics seen in up to 15% of children most likely to come into conflict with parental expectations involves irregular biologic rhythms, frequent withdrawal from new stimuli, slow adaptation, frequent negative mood, and high-intensity responding. Critically, the behavioral results of such mismatches likely do not reflect poor parenting or child psychopathology, and it is important to recognize, communicate, and help caregivers correct this.

Language Development and Effective Directive Delivery

Friman and Blum's (2002) discussion of language-based factors at play in problem behavior is particularly interesting and useful to practitioners. They point out, for example, that young children, particularly those under the age of 7, may not share the caregiver's conceptual ability to perceive sameness across situations, and in such cases caregivers' attempts to verbally assert sameness across situations (e.g., "How many times have I told you?") will fail to enlighten. The present moment inevitably varies in some ways (e.g., location, time of day, persons present) from the historical moment being verbally referenced by the caregiver and the child is not yet capable of perceiving the similarity of both moments. Doing so is made even more difficult for the child given the caregiver's expressed frustration and its predictable effects on the child's momentary ability to reason and desire to please. Caregivers should be urged to verbally stay within the present moment with their children, particularly with those younger than 7 years of age.

How directives are delivered impacts behavioral compliance as well. Clear, direct, and single-step directives, for example, are more likely to be followed than vaguely worded, indirect (e.g., issuing a request versus a command), and multistep directives. Importantly, older children who do not often immediately comply with caregiver directives and who "should know better" when given vaguely worded, indirect, and multistep directives likely do not have a track record of sufficient successful practice with more clearly communicated directives. Following directions represents a skill set to be shaped, not an instinctual behavior present at birth. Uncooperative children become more cooperative when caregivers switch to more effective delivery of directives, and more resulting cooperation in turn leads to more successful practice, helping to establish more instinctual cooperation in contexts including more vaguely worded, indirect, and multistep directives. More on effective directive delivery is found in Chapter 7.

Doing Versus Saying

Also discussed by Friman and Blum (2002) is an important distinction to be drawn between *saying* and *doing*, which is highly relevant for childrearing and for behavioral pediatrics. Likely all caregivers have experienced how their children are able to explain what they are to do – and when they don't do it, they are nonetheless perfectly able to describe what it was they were supposed to do. The clearest way of explaining this phenomenon is by pointing out that discussing behavior, and engaging in the behavior discussed, are two different skill sets. The ability to explain how to do something, we all know, does not automatically lead to the doing of it, let alone doing it to some standard. Caregivers are nonetheless prone to forget this in daily life and benefit from learning to have the child actually practice the desired behavior, not just listen or talk about it. Children need procedural coaching more than mere verbal prompting and lecturing. An example is helping the caregiver switch from asking a child with encopresis if he has to go, to physically (and supportively) escorting him to the potty when scheduled or otherwise indicated.

Repetition with Contrast

The final theoretical basis discussed by Friman and Blum (2002) has to do with how learning occurs, and while this material should not be news to behavior analysts, it is usually news to caregivers. A century of behavioral research supports the fundamental idea that a great deal of behavior occurs as a function of consequences (Friman, 2017; Skinner, 1938, 1953). Those consequences may be described in user-friendly terms as follows: Behavior can bring about pleasant or unpleasant outcomes for the child, and behavior that brings pleasant outcomes is likely to persist, whereas behavior that brings unpleasant outcomes is likely to decrease. And, critically, the learning of meaningful relationships between particular behaviors and outcomes is a function of experiential contrast between the consequences. The more contrast, the fewer repetitions of the association are required; the less contrast, the more repetitions will be required.

Friman and Blum's example of touching a flame in explaining experiential contrast is a good one: the contrast between 2,500°F and room temperature is enormous, and accidental contact with a 2,500-degree flame will very likely result in one-trial learning. Carrying this metaphor further, the reminders and warnings caregivers issue are operating at room temperature, offering little contrast and a high likelihood of desensitization to them. In the event caregivers wish to stop repeating themselves a thousand times, the consequence they engineer for their children should offer relatively more experiential contrast.

Corporal punishment has historically served a very strong contrast function, but the field of behavior analysis has endeavored to reduce its use by replacing it with less coercive alternatives that do not model aggression.

One such success story is the use of time-out (or, more exactly, *time-out from positive reinforcement*; see Chapter 7 for a review) as an alternative to corporal punishment. Implementation of time-out without a conceptual understanding of its purpose, however, renders it ineffective. Time-out as a consequence for attention-seeking problem behavior only works when the time-out condition 1) does not include the child experiencing contingent attention, and 2) there is sufficient contrast between the time-out and time-in conditions. For example, caregivers frequently deliver reprimands or lectures to a child during time-out, which lowers the metaphorical temperature of the consequence, in turn necessitating more repetitions of the procedure in order to achieve the desired effect. It is news to most caregivers that planned ignoring for behavior historically reinforced by attention, particularly when implemented consistently, can offer greater experiential contrast than anything else the caregiver can do in response to the behavior.

A Final Note

This chapter explored not only how to conceptualize problem behavior but also the larger systemic problem of a dominant behavioral healthcare model that is not very useful for understanding behavior. An alternative, more helpful model is advocated.

The progression of science can be a complicated matter given how systems develop around practices that for better or worse serve to maintain the status quo. Financial incentives and turf issues are classic features of such maintaining systems, and there appears no reason to believe behavioral healthcare is immune to such influences. The content of this chapter may be challenging for some readers but *fundamentally our differences are and must ultimately be about ideas, not about individuals*, as we not shy away from robust debate over those ideas.

Key Takeaways from this Chapter

- Mentalism is the underlying philosophy of much of modern behavioral healthcare involving the assumption that an inner metaphysical dimension, such as the mind, causes behavior. Functionalism, on the other hand, is the underlying philosophy of behavior analysis; the practice of primary care behavioral pediatrics assumes that behavior occurs as a function of circumstances.

- The dominant model in modern behavioral healthcare is the biomedical model. The biomedical model features the use of hypothetical constructs, which are speculative concepts invented to account for observable phenomena. Clinical diagnosis in behavioral healthcare represents the use of hypothetical constructs: specifically, hypothesized disease states that have yet to be empirically observed.

- The biomedical model has not been very successful from a scientific standpoint. To date, no biological variables have been identified which can help to verify the physical existence of any clinical diagnosis. The logical errors of reification, reductionism, circularity, argumentum ab auctoritate, argumentum ad populum, and the fundamental attribution error are easily committed when adhering to the biomedical model. No one *has* anything diagnosed although their topographical presentation might satisfy diagnostic criteria for a diagnosis.

- Research on the neurological causes of diagnostic conditions is correlational in nature and can therefore be misleading. There appears much more evidence to conclude that experience causes neurological changes than problem behavior is caused by pathological genetics, brain structure, or brain function.

- Behavior analysis is transdiagnostic and extradiagnostic in that it has broad applicability across diagnoses and may operate outside of the diagnostic classification system altogether. When collaborating with multidisciplinary professionals, behavior analysts are encouraged to view clinical diagnosis as verbal shorthand for topographical classes of behavior and to approach behavior consistently regardless of whether a class of behavior satisfies diagnostic criteria for a diagnosis.

- Temperamental factors and other sources of individual differences and their discordance with those of caregivers must be considered in case conceptualization and treatment. About 15% of children exhibit a particularly challenging cluster of behavioral tendencies involving irregular biologic rhythms, frequent withdrawal from new stimuli, slow adaptation, frequent negative mood, and high-intensity responding, which inevitably clash with caregiver expectations and lifestyle preferences.

- Caregivers should be encouraged to stay in the present moment verbally with their children, offer their children behavioral rehearsal of desired behavior in addition to simply talking about the desired behavior, and to present directives to their children that are clear, direct, and involve a single behavioral step at a time. Caregivers also require guidance in how to engineer behavioral contrast for their children. Desired behavior should be associated with pleasant outcomes whereas problem behavior should be associated with unpleasant outcomes. Caregivers should also be provided guidance on limits to those positive and negative consequences and on functional alternatives which may be more effective than what they have been using in terms of discipline methods.

References

Abramowitz, J. S. (2015). The biomedical model: Caveat emptor. *The Behavior Therapist, 38,* 169, 171–172.

American Academy of Pediatrics (2011). ADHD: Clinical practice guideline for the diagnosis, evaluation, and treatment of attention-deficit/hyperactivity disorder in children and adolescents. *Pediatrics, 128,* 1007–1022.

American Psychiatric Association (2022). *Diagnostic and statistical manual of mental disorders* (5th ed., text rev.). Author.

Ang, B., Horowitz, M., & Moncrieff, J. (2022). Is the chemical imbalance an "urban legend"? An exploration of the status of the serotonin theory of depression in the scientific literature. *SSM – Mental Health,* DOI: 10.1016/j.ssmmh.2022.100098

Baer, D. M., Wolf, M. M., & Risley, T. R. (1987). Some still-current dimensions of applied behavior analysis. *Journal of Applied Behavior Analysis, 20,* 313–327.

Barkley, R. A. (2018). Etiologies of ADHD. In R. A. Barkley (Ed.), *Attention-deficit hyperactivity disorder: A handbook for diagnosis and treatment* (4th ed., pp. 356–390). Guilford.

Baum, W. M. (2018). Multiscale behavior analysis and molar behaviorism: An overview. *Journal of the Experimental Analysis of Behavior, 110,* 302–322.

Bowden, M. G., Woodbury, M. L., & Duncan, P. W. (2013). Promoting neuroplasticity and recovery after stroke: Future directions for rehabilitation clinical trials. *Current Opinion in Neurology, 26,* 37–42.

Burgos, J. E., & Killeen, P. R. (2019). Suing for peace in the war against mentalism. *Perspectives on Behavior Science, 42,* 241–266.

Burton, R. A. (2013). *A skeptic's guide to the mind: What neuroscience can and cannot tell us about ourselves.* St. Martin's.

Castellanos, F. X., Giedd, J. N., Marsh, W. L., Hamburger, S. D., Vaituzis, A. C., Dickstein, D. P., Sarfatti, S. E., Vauss, Y. C., Snell, J. W., Lange, N., Kaysen, D., Krain, A. L., Ritchie, G. F., Rajapakse, J. C., & Rapoport, J. L. (1996). Quantitative brain magnetic resonance imaging in attention-deficit hyperactivity disorder. *Archives of General Psychiatry, 53,* 607–616.

Centers for Disease Control and Prevention (2022) *Attention-deficit/hyperactivity disorder.* CDC. www.cdc.gov/ncbddd/adhd/data.html

Christophersen, E. R. (1982). Incorporating behavioral pediatrics into primary care. *Pediatric Clinics of North America, 29,* 261–296.

Cooper, J. O., Heron, T. E., & Heward, W. L. (2020). *Applied behavior analysis* (3rd ed.). Pearson.

Deacon, B. J., & McKay, D. (2015). The biomedical model of psychological problems: A call for critical dialogue. *The Behavior Therapist, 38,* 231–235.

Dinsmoor, J. A. (1992). Setting the record straight. *American Psychologist, 47,* 1454–1463.

Edelbrock, C. S., & Costello, A. (1984). Structured psychiatric interviews for children and adolescents. In G. Goldstein & M. Hersen (Eds.), *Handbook of psychological assessment* (pp. 276–290). Pergamon.

Ehrlich, P. (2000). *Human natures: Genes, cultures, and the human prospect.* Island.

Evans, I. M. (2005). Applied behavior analysis. In M. Hersen, A. M. Gross, & R. S. Drabman (Eds.), *Encyclopedia of behavior modification and cognitive behavior therapy* (Vol. 2; pp. 666–674). Sage.

Fisher, W. W., Groff, R. A., & Roane, H. S. (2011). Applied behavior analysis: History, philosophy, principles, and basic methods. In W. W. Fisher, C. C. Piazza, & H. S. Roane (Eds.), *Handbook of applied behavior analysis* (pp. 3–13). Guilford.

Fraley, L. E., & Vargas, E. A. (1986). Separate disciplines: The study of behavior and the study of the psyche. *The Behavior Analyst, 9,* 47–59.

Fredrick, L. D., & Hummel, J. H. (2004). Reviewing the outcomes and principles of effective instruction. In D. J. Moran & R. W. Malott (Eds.), *Evidence-based educational methods* (pp. 9–22). Academic.

Friman, P. C. (2017). You are in the way! Opening lines of transmission for Skinner's view of behavior. *The Behavior Analyst, 40,* 173–177.

Friman, P. C. (2021). There is no such thing as a bad boy: The circumstances view of problem behavior. *Journal of Applied Behavior Analysis, 54,* 636–653.

Friman, P. C., & Blum, N. J. (2002). Primary care behavioral pediatrics. In M. Hersen & W. Sledge (Eds.), *Encyclopedia of psychotherapy* (pp. 379–399). Academic.

Gaser, C., & Schlaug, G. (2003). Brain structures differ between musicians and non-musicians. *Journal of Neuroscience, 23,* 9240–9245, doi: 10.1523/JNEUROSCI.23-27-09240.2003

Glenn, S. S., Ellis, J., & Greenspoon, J. (1992). On the revolutionary nature of the operant as a unit of behavioral selection. *American Psychologist, 47,* 1329–1336.

Gotzsche, P. C., & Healy, D. (2022). Restoring the two pivotal fluoxetine trials in children and adolescents with depression. *International Journal of Risk and Safety in Medicine, 33,* 385–408.

Hayes, S. C., Sanford, B. T., & Feeney, T. K. (2015). Using the functional and contextual approach of modern evolution science to direct thinking about psychopathology. *The Behavior Therapist, 38,* 222–227.

Iuculano, T., Rosenberg-Lee, M., Richardson, J., Tenison, C., Fuchs, L., Supekar, K., & Menon, V. (2015). Cognitive tutoring induces widespread neuroplasticity and remediates brain function in children with mathematical learning disabilities. *Nature Communications, 6,* 8453, DOI: 10.1038/ncomms9453

Johnston, J. M., Pennypacker, H. S., & Green, G. (2020). *Strategies and tactics of behavioral research and practice* (4th ed.). Routledge.

Kates, W. R., Mostofsky, S. H., Zimmerman, A. W., Mazzocco, M. M., Landa, R., Warsofsky, W. E., Kaufmann, W. E., & Reiss, A. L. (1998). Neuroanatomical and neurocognitive differences in a pair of monozygotic twins discordant for strictly defined autism. *Annals of Neurology, 43,* 782–791.

Kays, J. L., Hurley, R. A., & Taber, K. H. (2012). The dynamic brain: Neuroplasticity and mental health. *Journal of Neuropsychiatry and Clinical Neurosciences, 24,* 118–124.

Kirsch, I. (2010). *The emperor's new drugs: Exploding the antidepressant myth.* Basic.

Kirsch, I., Moore, T. J., Scoboria, A., & Nicholls, S. S. (2002). The emperor's new drugs: An analysis of antidepressant medication data submitted to the U.S. Food and Drug Administration. *Prevention & Treatment*, https://psycnet.apa.org/fulltext/2002-14079-003.pdf

Kleim, J. A., & Jones, T. A. (2008). Principles of experience-dependent neural plasticity: Implications for rehabilitation after brain damage. *Journal of Speech, Language, and Hearing Research, 51*, S225–S239. Downloaded from: https://pubs.asha.org73.49.208.109.

Kolb, B., & Gibb, R. (2008). Principles of neuroplasticity and behavior. In D. T. Stuss, G. Winocur, & I. H. Robertson (Eds.), *Cognitive neurorehabilitation: Evidence and application* (2nd ed., pp. 6–21). Cambridge.

Lacasse, J. R., & Leo, J. (2005). Serotonin and depression: A disconnect between the advertisements and the scientific literature. *PLoS Med 2(12)*: e392.

Lacasse, J. R., & Leo, J. (2015). Antidepressants and the chemical imbalance theory of depression: A reflection and update of the discourse. *The Behavior Therapist, 38*, 206–213.

Lovasz, N., & Slaney, K. (2013). What makes a hypothetical construct "hypothetical"? Tracing the origins and uses of the "hypothetical construct" concept in psychological science. *New Ideas in Psychology, 31.* DOI: 10.1016/j.newideapsych.2011.02.005

MacCorquodale, K., & Meehl, P. E. (1948). On a distinction between hypothetical constructs and intervening variables. *Psychological Review, 55*, 95–107.

Mansson, K. N. T., Salami, A., Frick, A., Carlbring, P., Andersson, G., Furmark, T., & Boraxbekk, C. J. (2016). Neuroplasticity in response to cognitive behavior therapy for social anxiety disorder. *Translational Psychiatry, 6*, e727, DOI 10.1038/tp.2015.218

Molfese, D. L. (2011). Advancing neuroscience through epigenetics: Molecular mechanisms of learning and memory. *Developmental Neuropsychology, 36*, 810–827.

Moncrieff, J. Cooper, R. E., Stockmann, T., Amendola, S., Hengartner, M. P., & Horowitz, M. A. (2022). The serotonin theory of depression: A systematic umbrella review of the evidence. *Molecular Psychiatry*, doi: 10.1038/s41380-022-01661-0

Moore, J. (1995). Radical behaviorism and the subjective-objective distinction. *The Behavior Analyst, 18*, 33–49.

Moore, J. (2003). Behavior, analysis, mentalism, and the path to social justice. *The Behavior Analyst, 26*, 181–193.

Mychasiuk, R. (2015). Epigenetics of brain plasticity and behavior. In J. D. Wright (Ed.), *International encyclopedia of the social & behavioral sciences* (2nd ed., Vol. 7, pp. 848–851). Elsevier.

National Institute for Direct Instruction (n.d.). *Project follow through.* www.nifdi.org/what-is-di/project-follow-through

National Institutes of Health (2013). *Harnessing neuroplasticity for behavior change*: Meeting report. https://commonfund.nih.gov/sites/default/files/FINAL_SOBC_Sept_2013_neuroplasticity_report_REV_2-25-14v2.pdf

National Institutes of Health (2013). *Harnessing neuroplasticity for behavior change*: Meeting report. https://commonfund.nih.gov/sites/default/files/FINAL_SOBC_Sept_2013_neuroplasticity_report_REV_2-25-14v2.pdf

Nikolas, M. A., & Burt, A. (2010). Genetic and environmental influences on ADHD symptom dimensions of inattention and hyperactivity: A meta-analysis. *Journal of Abnormal Psychology, 119*, 1–17.

Popper, K. (1959). *The logic of scientific discovery.* Hutchinson.

Rosenberg, A., & McIntyre, L. (2020). *Philosophy of science: A contemporary introduction* (4th ed.). Routledge.

Schlinger, H. D. (1995). *A behavior analytic view of child development.* Plenum.

Schlinger, H. D. (2015). Behavior, analysis, and behavioral neuroscience. *Frontiers in Human Neuroscience,* DOI 10.3389/fnhum.2015.00210

Scull, A. (2021). American psychiatry in the new millennium: A critical appraisal. *Psychological Medicine, 51,* 2762–2770.

Shermer, M. (2002). *Why people believe weird things: Pseudoscience, superstition, and other confusions of our time.* Owl.

Simos, P. G., Fletcher, J. M., Bergmann, E., Breier, J. I., Foorman, B. R., Castillo, E. M., Davis, R. N., Fitzgerald, M., & Papanicolaou, A. C. (2002). Dyslexia-specific brain activation profile becomes normal following successful remedial training. *Neurology, 58,* 1203–1213.

Simons, R. L., & Klopack, E. T. (2015). Invited address: "'The times they are a-changin'": Gene expression, neuroplasticity, and developmental research. *Journal of Youth and Adolescence, 44,* 573–580.

Skinner, B. F. (1938). *The behavior of organisms: An experimental analysis.* Appleton-Century-Crofts.

Skinner, B. F. (1953). *Science and human behavior.* Free Press.

Thomas, A., & Chess, S. (1977). *Temperament and development.* Brunner/Mazel.

Uher, R., & Rutter, M. (2012). Basing psychiatric classification on scientific foundation: Problems and prospects. *International Review of Psychiatry, 24,* 591–605.

van Ewijk, H., Heslenfeld, D. J., Zwiers, M. P., Buitelaar, J. K., & Oosterlaan, J. (2012). Diffusion tensor imaging in attention deficit/hyperactivity disorder: A systematic review and meta-analysis. *Neuroscience and Biobehavioral Review, 36,* 1093–1106.

Whitaker, R. (2015). Anatomy of an epidemic: The history and science of a failed paradigm of care. *The Behavior Therapist, 38,* 192–198.

Woodworth, R. S. (1929). *Psychology* (rev. ed.). Holt.

Woollett, K., & Maguire, E. A. (2011). Acquiring "the Knowledge" of London's layout drives structural brain changes. *Current Biology, 21,* 2109–2114.

World Health Organization (2019). *International statistical classification of diseases and related health problems* (11th ed.). https://icd.who.int/

Assessment Methods   **3**

The behavior analyst practicing primary care behavioral pediatrics will be familiar with assessment concepts, approaches, and methods common to applied behavior-analytic practice but should also be reasonably familiar and conversant with common practices in traditional behavioral healthcare. Demonstrating an understanding of more traditional assessment methods potentially makes the behavior analyst a more valuable collaborator and, in some ways, may deepen the well of data from which the behavior analyst may draw insight. As such, this chapter first endeavors to offer the behavior analyst a primer of the work commonly done by traditional behavioral healthcare practitioners. From there, we explore the assessment methods most relevant to the practice of behavioral pediatrics.

Assessment in Traditional Behavioral Healthcare

As observed by Vlaeyen and colleagues (2020) regarding mental health treatment, "Psychology is the science of the individual, yet the bulk of available research data is derived from groups" (p. 659). Clinical assessment in psychology similarly tends to be *nomothetic* rather than *idiographic* in nature; clients are typically evaluated as to their relative position within a larger group instead of as individuals with their own unique learning histories and present circumstances. It is also consistent with the philosophy of mentalism and the biomedical model of mental illness.

DOI: 10.4324/9781003371281-4

Traditional assessment stands upon four pillars: interviews, observations, standardized norm-referenced testing, and use of "informal" assessment procedures (Sattler, 2001), with the latter including record review, journaling and other anecdotal recording, and criterion-referenced testing (i.e., written tests or other tasks which assess skill mastery). The pièce de résistance here is what psychologists think of as "formal" procedures, the standardized norm-referenced testing exemplified by intelligence, or IQ (intelligence quotient), testing. *Standardized* means the test is administered the same way to every individual, and *norm-referenced* means the individual's performance is statistically compared to that of others. IQ testing involves administering a series of subtests to children, each yielding raw scores which are then statistically compared to how other same-age children have scored, which, in turn, yields scaled scores per subtest. These scaled scores then are statistically summarized by a set of standard scores, locating the child's performance along a bell curve, or normal distribution. These resulting scores reflect hypothetical constructs such as, in the case of the Wechsler Intelligence Scale for Children, Fifth Edition, verbal comprehension, visual-spatial reasoning, fluid reasoning, working memory, processing speed, and general intelligence. A Full Scale IQ standard score falling between 90 and 109 means the child demonstrates average intellectual ability. A Processing Speed standard score of 70 means the child's visuomotor speed is slower than 98% of same-age peers. Norm-referenced achievement tests, such as the Woodcock-Johnson, work the same way.

Neuropsychological test batteries include much more than just an IQ and achievement test and therefore yield dozens of specific (typically norm-referenced) scores the overall pattern of which is held to offer unique insights about the child. The ultimate goal for psychological and neuropsychological evaluations is to arrive at a diagnostic impression and a list of recommendations based upon that impression. Individual strengths and weaknesses are highlighted and need or eligibility for certain accommodations and remedial programs or therapies is examined and asserted. Concern exists, however, over the usefulness of neuropsychological testing in, for example, the diagnosis of ADHD (Solanto, 2018; Willcutt, 2018). Furthermore, findings and recommendations from batteries of norm-referenced tests are rarely function-based. Some psychologists who are more behaviorally trained may include a functional behavior assessment (FBA) section and resulting function-based recommendations. Otherwise, such tests and assessment batteries, from a behavior-analytic perspective, can be useful at least from the standpoint of identifying problem topographies and incongruities between skill repertoires and task demands. They also help determine eligibility for special school programs and funding (e.g., special education under a learning disability classification, or a gifted classroom).

Behavioral rating scales, such as the Child Behavior Checklist and Conners Rating Scale, involve soliciting informant ratings commonly along a three- or four-point Likert-scale on a large number of items. Many of these rating scales solicit self-ratings from the child client as well. Ratings are scored against a comparison group, and the results, like formal testing discussed above, inform of the amount of deviance from the average on a number of hypothetical constructs. Such instruments are purported to assist with clinical diagnosis. Again, from a behavior-analytic perspective, such data can be useful; scores from different informants can reveal who may be struggling the most with the child, how, and to what extent.

Projective testing includes, for example, the Rorschach Inkblot Test, and a number of drawing tasks such as House-Tree-Person. The concept of *projection* in mental measurement has been described as "the tendency of people to be influenced by their needs, interests, and overall psychological organization in the cognitive translation or interpretation of perceptual inputs whenever the stimulus field included some ambiguity" (Exner, 1993, p. 15) and it is argued that these tests are useful in "providing access to unconscious material that the person would otherwise be unable or un-willing to communicate" (Hunsley *et al.*, 2015, p. 60, citing Handler, 1985). Those who use projectives are attempting to access something they suspect is underlying the observed and reported problems. Projective testing is however rife with problems with reliability and validity (Hunsley *et al.*, 2015; Lilienfeld, Wood & Garb, 2000) and from a functionalist perspective is particularly vestigial, rooted in the prehistory of our collective attempts to understand why people do what they do. It nevertheless remains quite popular among psychologists; a recent survey (Mihura *et al.*, 2022) found that two-thirds of psychologists in the US continue to use the Rorschach.

Some psychologists who conduct psychological evaluations choose to specialize in evaluation to the exclusion of treatment. Assessment is all they do. Other psychologists and most master's-level therapists do not offer psychological evaluation services at all and a client may receive a course of therapy from start to finish without ever undergoing a psychological eva-luation. And then there are large nonprofit agencies known for requiring a psychological evaluation on every new client before treatment, whether indicated or not. Thus, in the world of traditional behavioral healthcare, there is either a lot of assessment, or very little, if any, before treatment begins, and the relevance of assessment to treatment can be unclear.

What about after treatment begins? Continuous measurement during the course of treatment, or collecting data in any form, is rare among psychologists (Phelps, Eisman, & Kohout, 1998). Those who do employ outcome measures are in the minority and tend to be the newest to the profession and the most behaviorally trained (Bickman *et al.*, 2000; Hatfield & Ogles, 2004; Phelps, Eisman, & Kohout, 1998).

Assessment in Behavioral Pediatrics

Assessment in behavioral pediatrics is *idiographic* rather than *nomothetic*. While developmental expectations are taken into account, the behavior of clients and their family members is viewed as a product of their own unique learning histories and present circumstances. Assessment is not based around hypothetical constructs but around the circumstances in which behavior occurs and does not occur, around what habits the child has been practicing, and what habits might instead be practiced that would work better for all involved. As discussed in Chapter 2, the problem is not assumed to be inside the person. Assessment in behavioral pediatrics is focused on the successful prediction and influence of behavior, seeking to know which functional relationships to leverage, and to determine what new behaviors to teach to whom that would result in effective, efficient, durable, and socially valid treatment.

If, for example, problem behavior usually occurs when a child is asked to relinquish his gaming system, rather than viewing this behavior as a symptom of a disease entity called *oppositional defiant disorder*, perhaps the timing of the request or the timing of access to gaming could be altered to change the outcome. If siblings tend to fight over a mutually preferred item, perhaps the siblings could be taught conflict prevention skills such as appropriately manding for the item. If a child doesn't know the socially appropriate response to the situation, perhaps we can teach it, and engineer the environment to respond well to its practice so the fragile new skill is maintained. That new skill takes the place of the problem behavior the old situation tended to elicit. Assessment directly informs our case formulation and guides our treatment, and helps maintain the quality of ongoing services per case. Again, this approach is useful regardless of clinical diagnosis and in fact requires no diagnosis at all.

This chapter is not intended to replace the available behavioral measurement textbooks (e.g., Bailey & Burch, 2018; Johnston, Pennypacker, & Green, 2020) but instead endeavors to offer an overview of the various approaches and methods of assessment relevant to the practice of behavioral pediatrics. Topics covered here include taking the history, conducting observations, functional behavior assessment, reinforcer assessment, social validity, and progress monitoring.

Getting The History: Questionnaire, Record Review, and Interview

Obtaining a comprehensive history (and doing so efficiently) is perhaps best achieved via a combination of questionnaire, record review, and interview. The history questionnaire is a particularly important clinical tool, allowing the collection of a wide array of information even before families arrive for the initial appointment. Some practitioners may wish to collect this information in person, however, or to assign such duties to well-trained RBTs. In any case, information solicited via questionnaire will help give shape to the clinical interview. This questionnaire should cover the following categories of information (for a sample history questionnaire, see Schroeder & Smith-Boydston, 2017):

- Demographics, including marital status, caregiver occupations, and identification of everyone living in the home
- Religious affiliations and other cultural information
- Current sources of stress for each family member
- Physicians and other providers historically and currently involved in the child's care
- School and academic history
- Strengths and interests
- Trauma history
- Friendships and socialization
- Birth history
- Early developmental history
- Historical and current medical concerns (including major illnesses, injuries, surgeries, hospitalizations, and history of head trauma)
- Behavioral health history, including previous providers, description of treatment, and perceived effectiveness; also, medication history and prescribing physicians
- Allied pediatric therapy (occupational, physical, and speech) history
- Allergies
- Last physical exam and vision and hearing exams

- Family medical and mental health history
- How each caregiver recalls being raised and whether they have fond memories of their childhood
- Cooperation screening: compliance rate and toleration level for denial of wishes
- Multiple choice checklist listing all manner of common problems of childhood
- Total screen time on weekdays and weekends, devices used, and rough percentage of gaming versus educational use
- Bedtime and sleep health and habits
- Anything else the caregiver wishes to share

I prefer to have caregivers complete the history questionnaire and upload relevant records through a secure online client portal as part of the client registration process and to meet caregivers without the child for the initial appointment either in person or via telehealth to carefully review and discuss the history without distraction or self-editing on anyone's part. This first appointment with caregivers also allows an opportunity to build rapport and provide an overview of the approach. It is also an opportunity to instill hope and secure commitments to robust collaborative communication and high treatment adherence.

Records shared by caregivers in behavioral pediatrics tend to include psychoeducational and neuropsychological evaluation reports and various school records, including grade reports and anecdotal notes from the classroom describing problem behavior. The vast majority of the latter describe problem behavior but lack helpful contextual information; early correspondence with the teacher for insight as to context can prove critically important in understanding and solving the challenges described.

The initial clinical interview allows the practitioner to fill in any blanks left by the questionnaire and record review, and to explore caregivers' attributions about the problem behavior. Asking caregivers how they were raised and whether they have fond memories of their childhoods can offer insight as to whether they may be overcorrecting in their management approach; a caregiver who as a child was raised under a strict authoritarian approach, for example, may be engaging in rule-governed permissiveness (e.g., "I'm not going to raise my children the way I was raised"), not realizing that the most effective management approach may lie somewhere between these two poles of the child management continuum. Building the historical timeline and trajectory of problem behaviors is also a critical step.

Observation

My typical practice is to devote an hour-long session to observation. The family immediately enters a play environment with age-appropriate toys and activities. I strive to establish myself as a reinforcer, placing on the child no demands for the first third of the one-hour appointment. Interactions between parent and child are sampled. In the next step, a series of demands are presented, based on information collected to this point and aimed at developing treatment goals. Compliance rate, toleration of frustration, denial, and delay, verbal manding repertoire, social and emotional reciprocity, coachability, and task persistence are sampled. Observation may be done in the home or classroom, on the playground, or in clinic, and caregivers may be invited to capture some video of representative moments in the home and send them along for review. Sampling not only the settings and situations of concern but also when and where things go well can be informative. Caregivers may be asked how they typically handle certain situations, to get a sense of whether they use a basic repertoire of teaching skills or inadvertently reinforce extinction bursts.

Technology has increasingly played a role in assessment efforts. Originally dubbed ecological momentary assessment by Stone and Shiffman (1994), modern apps may now prompt the client or caregiver to record an observation at certain intervals, or at certain times of day; providers can often access and review the data before the next appointment. It is likely that data of this sort would be more reliable than retrospective self-report in session. If no app exists for a particular clinical purpose along these lines, the provider may assist the client or caregiver in setting regular alerts on their smartphones and record the data on an app such as Apple's Notes.

Functional Behavior Assessment

The core of behavior-analytic practice is FBA. As such, an historical and procedural overview is offered here. The point of FBA is ultimately to identify what to teach the child and caregivers to do instead and what to change about the social and physical environment to in turn bring about the desired change in behavior. Doing so allows treatment effectiveness to reach 90% and higher (Fisher *et al.*, 2023).

Behavior modification of decades past involved the application of arbitrary "positive" and "negative" consequences contingent upon certain behaviors with the intent of overpowering natural sources of reinforcement for problem behavior (Hanley, Iwata, & McCord, 2003; Mace, 1994). This was form over function. Critical conceptual and procedural refinements were introduced in 1982 by Iwata and colleagues: basing treatment on assessed and hypothesized behavioral function. By analyzing the contingencies maintaining problem behavior, individually tailored behavior change programs become possible. Such efforts are more effective and arguably more considerate and humane (Hanley, 2012).

FBA methodology was developed in attempts to determine the function of high-rate, high-intensity problem behavior of clients with severe impairments, a population representing about 90% of published research employing FBA (Hanley, Iwata, & McCord, 2003; see also Beavers, Iwata, & Lerman, 2013, and Melanson & Fahmie, 2023). In time, the use of this methodology was extended to typically developing children (Gardner et al., 2012; see also Wacker, Schieltz, & Romani, 2015).

FBA is comprised of three procedural components: indirect assessment, descriptive assessment, and functional analysis. Indirect assessment methods include reports from various parties; interviews, questionnaires, and rating scales are employed. Structured interviews (e.g., Bailey & Pyles, 1989; Hanley, 2012; Kern et al., 1995; O'Neill et al., 1997; Rolider & Van Houten, 1993) and screener instruments (e.g., Durand & Crimmins, 1992; Iwata & DeLeon, 1996; Lewis, Scott, & Sugai, 1994; Paclawskyj et al., 2000; Wieseler et al., 1985) have been made available through the years. Indirect assessment allows for generating tentative functional hypotheses that inform preliminary treatment recommendations. No research has validated the use of indirect assessment alone, and it is not recommended for use in isolation (Hanley et al., 2014; Neef & Peterson, 2007).

A descriptive assessment combines indirect assessment with direct observation of the behavior in question in the context in which it typically occurs. Neef and Peterson (2007) list scatterplot analysis and ABC continuous and narrative recording as variations of descriptive analysis, all geared to reveal patterns of behavior-context relationships that might lead to the formation of functional hypotheses. Scatterplots help uncover temporal patterns that can be more closely examined later by other means. ABC (antecedent-behavior-consequence) continuous recording refers to simple frequency count, partial interval, or momentary time sampling recording over a selected interval of time during which the problem behavior typically occurs. An efficient method of data collection might involve a coded data sheet already developed based upon initial indirect assessment findings. A less formal, less rigorous technique is ABC narrative recording, which essentially involves writing down the antecedent conditions and apparent consequences whenever the target behavior occurs; Neef and Peterson recommend this only for collecting preliminary information leading to more formal data collection or functional analysis.

The third procedural component, functional analysis, was originally introduced conceptually by Skinner (1953) and decades later came to refer to the manipulation of antecedent and consequent variables and observing the effect on the behavior in question. We are essentially running an experiment here, testing the functional hypotheses formed via descriptive assessment. Iwata and colleagues' 1982 article details an early example of this experimental approach: To examine sources of reinforcement maintaining self-injury, they designed four alternating conditions for each of nine children with developmental disabilities which included contingent attention, contingent escape, alone, and unstructured play, with the latter representing a control condition in which toys and other fun activities were available, appropriate behavior was praised, inappropriate behavior was ignored, and no task demands were presented. An alternating treatments design was employed to determine which condition evoked the most problem behavior for each child. They found that for six children, the problem behavior was consistently associated with a specific condition; while this was an important finding, another important finding was that problem behavior—here, self-injury—can serve multiple functions for each child depending upon the immediate circumstances.

The "Iwata model," or extended functional analysis, has been a mainstay of applied behavior analysis and such methodology has been refined through the years (see Betz & Fisher, 2011, Call, Scheithauer, & Mevers, 2017; Contreras *et al.*, 2023, and Hanley, Iwata, & McCord, 2003, for reviews) with a later procedural variation known as *brief functional analysis* showing up in the literature in the 1990s (e.g., Cooper *et al.*, 1990; Cooper *et al.*, 1992; Northup *et al.*, 1991; Northup *et al.*, 1994). Brief functional analysis tests a minimum of two conditions, and the single-subject experimental design can be ABAB or reversal, alternating treatments or multielement, or pairwise (sequentially pairing each test condition with the control condition). Test conditions can include contingent attention, escape, tangibles (material or edible), automatic reinforcement/sensory input, and others. Some have drawn a distinction between socially mediated and non-socially mediated sources of positive and negative reinforcement (e.g., Cipani, 2018; Miltenberger, 2016). The duration of each functional analysis is determined by however long it takes to obtain useful information. Brief functional analyses have been successfully conducted over only several days, with two or fewer observations for each test condition (see Northup *et al.*, 1991). Sessions can be brief (e.g., within a single 5-minute session) or longer (e.g., longer sessions across multiple weeks); Wallace and Iwata (1999) reported no difference between 5-minute and 15-minute sessions in terms of outcome, and Hanley and colleagues' (2003) review found 10-minute sessions to be most common.

In efforts to further improve assessment efficiency, Hanley (2012; see also Jessel, Hanley, & Ghaemmaghami, 2016) proposed a streamlined process involving an open-ended interview (versus use of closed-ended rating scales; see his 2012 article for his interview form), a brief observation, the forming of functional hypotheses, and testing them by first engineering a control condition in which the assumed reinforcer is made freely available, followed by a test condition in which the assumed reinforcer is withheld at fixed intervals (e.g., every 30 seconds) and returned contingent upon the problem behavior (e.g., Hanley *et al.*, 2014; the sequence of the control and test conditions may be reversed in order to obtain a baseline in the presence of the controlling contingency). This is then followed by the control condition to examine whether the problem behavior is reduced along relevant parameters by the removal of that contingency. In colloquial terms, this process is intended to see whether we can reliably "turn the behavior on and off," as Hanley describes it. If we can, then we have identified the function and understand the behavior.

Functional analysis may be unnecessary in cases involving restricted operants (behaviors evoked under highly specific conditions; Hanley, 2012). These may include noncompliance, food refusal, and behavior interfering with sleep onset and maintenance. In such cases in which the function is fairly predictable, a rough baseline can be established via interview, and response to prescribed behavioral treatment can serve the purposes of analysis. Behavioral pediatric practice encounters a great deal of problem behavior of this kind; in day-to-day work, descriptive assessment alone may suffice, with functional analysis conducted when indicated.

FBA should not be limited to client behavior. Problem behavior often trains caregivers, siblings, teachers, and classmates to avoid evoking it, and that avoidance becomes negatively reinforced (Carr, Taylor, & Robison, 1991). Seeking help from a behavioral healthcare provider often represents an endpoint of such an adaptation process. Behavioral pediatrics therefore typically implies assessing and treating caregiver behavior too. This understanding is the essence of prescriptive behavioral treatment detailed in Chapter 4, and the heart of the recommendations for ensuring caregiver adherence discussed in Chapter 11.

Reinforcer Identification

Whereas FBA seeks to identify inadvertent sources of reinforcement for problem behavior, reinforcer identification deals with efforts to identify potential reinforcers to be intentionally offered contingent upon desired behavior. In designing incentivization programs for children as part of a comprehensive treatment plan, a key component is the reward chosen by the designer. Those who are not behavior analysts are likely to view "rewards" (e.g., stickers, points, money, candy) as examples of positive reinforcers; behavior analysts remain curious as to what *acts* as a reinforcer, regardless of what might be expected to act as a reinforcer. It is therefore important to proactively assess what rewards may indeed serve as positive reinforcers in a given case, and to be aware that this can change over time.

Preference assessment methodology was developed decades ago and refined over the years to help with reward selection (Fisher *et al.*, 1992; Hanley *et al.*, 2003; Pace *et al.*, 1985; Roane *et al.*, 1998). Most study participants were diagnosed with developmental disabilities; with these children, it wasn't as simple as asking them what they wanted to work toward. Typically developing children may be asked directly, but their answers do not always align with their observed preferences in contexts of interest (Northup *et al.*, 1996). Caregiver and teacher reports may also be unreliable (Favell & Cannon, 1976; Fantuzzo *et al.*, 1991).

What works best? The more data, the better, it appears. Generally speaking, the combination of self-report and caregiver-report (and teacher-report) with direct assessment seems to be the most reliable method for assessing reinforcer preference (Cote *et al.*, 2007; Fisher *et al.*, 1996). For more information, the reader is referred to Saini and colleagues' (2021) recent chapter on stimulus preference assessment and reinforcer identification.

Social Validity

Wolf's 1978 paper on social validity describes in amusing detail how a hard science of behavior came to unapologetically include soft, subjective measures. It is the story of an epiphany that the applied scientist cannot know best and that the customer is always right. Modern ABA solicits and incorporates input from the client, family, and others, tailoring treatment to match goals and preferences, adjusting procedures along the way to optimize and maintain acceptability and treatment adherence, and learning from feedback at case closure to inform future practice. Social validity as a complementary measure of effectiveness was, in fact, added to the *current dimensions* of ABA (i.e., applied, behavioral, analytic, technological, conceptually systematic, effective, and durable; Baer, Wolf, & Risley, 1968) by Baer and colleagues (1987). Importantly, Wolf (1978) explains that the primary reason Watson and Skinner rejected subjective measurement was not subjectivity, per se, but rather "the inappropriate causal roles that hypothetical internal variables, subjectively reported, were playing in social science" (p. 213). Subjective measurement for social validity purposes is not seeking an inner causal agent, but collecting data that are not otherwise observable, in order to ensure we are serving our clients and society well.

Common and Lane (2017) offer a wonderful overview of four usual methods of social validity assessment: interviews, self-report rating scales, direct assessment (e.g., preference assessment), and external evaluation (e.g., using content experts). Competent behavioral healthcare services involve comprehensive interviews of clients and caregivers, and other stakeholders may be interviewed as well. Direct assessment includes preference assessment, normative comparison, and sustained use (Common & Lane, 2017). Normative comparison involves the ascertainment of typical levels of performance of peers within the target setting, for example, for use in goal setting for the client. Sustained use refers to whether caregivers and others continue to implement the treatment over time, which may be taken as an indicator of acceptability. Lastly, external evaluation involves asking content experts, such as physicians or teachers, to rate the acceptability of a treatment or goal.

Baseline Establishment and Progress Monitoring

Establishing a baseline, followed by repeated measurement, is a hallmark of behavior-analytic work. Because behavioral pediatrics typically involves consultation with caregivers over a relatively brief period, direct observation or objective measurement may not be needed. The rigorous, objective behavioral assessment required for work with severely impaired individuals, or for publication in a peer-reviewed journal, is not required in behavioral pediatrics given the nature of the population served and behavior addressed. However, repeated measures in some form should inform treatment.

Barlow, Hayes, and Nelson, in their classic 1984 measurement textbook, recommended starting systematic measurement as early as possible, using as many measures as available and practicable (only some of which may be retained over time, based on their ultimate relevance to the case), and taking measures as frequently as possible without it being too intrusive. Baseline may be taken until the degree and sources of variability of behavior are discernible; protracted instability in the data might prompt a closer look at the sources of variability or the sampling interval chosen.

With procedural efficiency and social validity in mind, I routinely by Session 3 negotiate a list of treatment goals and establish a baseline for each goal in the form of Likert ratings from 0 (as bad as can be) to 10 (not perfect, but no concern) from caregivers. Frequency counts and percentages of opportunities are also solicited based upon the nature of the goals (e.g., aggressive behavior, noncompliance). Baseline can be established via observation or retrospection and may only be one or two data points per goal. Ratings are then solicited at the beginning of each subsequent session to allow for the examination of treatment effects on targeted behaviors as well as on problem behaviors not yet directly treated. These Likert ratings and other data collected are graphed and shared with the caregiver for visual inspection, analysis, and discussion. Improvements in level and trend present opportunities for reinforcement of caregiver treatment adherence, whereas no or little improvement may occasion problem solving of low treatment adherence or a necessary revisiting of the case formulation or treatment procedures selected. The graphical display of the data may be basic, as in an AB design, or more granular, separating each treatment phase by treatment component. A followup phase, typically three months out, is reflected in a single data point per goal.

Ultimately, practitioners have many options for measuring progress and for representing that progress graphically. The key is to collect the data and allow those data to inform decision making throughout treatment.

Key Takeaways from this Chapter

- Clinical assessment in traditional behavioral healthcare is nomothetic rather than idiographic; clients are evaluated as members of a reference group, instead of as individuals with unique learning histories and present circumstances. Assessment in behavioral pediatrics is idiographic rather than nomothetic; while developmental expectations are taken into account, the behavior of clients and their family members is viewed as a product of unique learning histories and present circumstances.
- History-taking is best done with a combination of questionnaires, a record review, and an interview of the child and caregivers. Information from the questionnaires and record review gives shape to the interview.

Observation offers critical additional insight and may be supplemented with video clips shared by caregivers.

- The heart of behavior-analytic practice is functional behavior assessment (FBA). FBA represents contingency analysis, or consideration of environmental conditions that make behavior more or less likely. Its three components are indirect assessment (use of interviews, questionnaires, and rating scales), descriptive assessment (indirect assessment plus observation), and functional analysis (indirect and descriptive assessment, plus active experimentation with antecedent and consequent variables). Procedural variations of functional analysis have been developed over time to attain greater efficiency.

- While the concepts underlying the traditional three components of FBA are critical for success in the practice of behavioral pediatrics, the functional analysis component is not as necessary with the largely neurotypical primary care pediatric population. Clients typically have greater verbal competence and may be queried directly, and the problem behaviors encountered involve more restricted operants, or behaviors with fairly predictable functions, evoked under highly specific conditions. The behavior of caregivers and others in the child's life is also subject to FBA.

- Reinforcer identification, or preference assessment, is the systematic assessment of current reinforcers for individual clients. Verbally competent clients may be asked directly what they prefer; however, children's verbal responses outside of the context of interest, as well as the reports of caregivers and teachers, may be unreliable. A combination of interviews and direct assessment likely offers the most reliable information.

- Social validity as a complementary, subjective measure of effectiveness was added to the *current dimensions* of ABA in 1987. Measuring social validity helps to ensure we are best serving our client's needs and those of caregivers and other stakeholders.

- Rigorous objective measurement is typically not required for treatment success in behavioral pediatrics given the nature of the population served and behavior addressed; nonetheless, continuous measurement in some form represents an essential feature of daily practice.

References

Baer, D. M., Wolf, M. M., & Risley, T. R. (1968). Some current dimensions of applied behavior analysis. *Journal of Applied Behavior Analysis, 1*, 91–97.

Baer, D. M., Wolf, M. M., & Risley, T. R. (1987). Some still-current dimensions of applied behavior analysis. *Journal of Applied Behavior Analysis, 20*, 313–327.

Bailey, J. S., & Burch, M. R. (2018). *Research methods in applied behavior analysis* (2nd ed.). Routledge.

Bailey, J. S., & Pyles, D. A. M. (1989). Behavioral diagnostics. In E. Cipani (Ed.), *The treatment of severe behavior disorders: Behavior analysis approach* (pp. 85–107). American Association on Mental Retardation.

Barlow, D. H., Hayes, S. C., & Nelson, R. O. (1984). *The scientist practitioner: Research and accountability in clinical and educational settings.* Allyn and Bacon.

Beavers, G. A., Iwata, B. A., & Lerman, D. C. (2013). Thirty years of research on the functional analysis of problem behavior. *Journal of Applied Behavior Analysis, 46,* 1–21.

Betz, A. M., & Fisher, W. W. (2011). Functional analysis: History and methods. In W. W. Fisher, C. C. Piazza, & H. S. Roane (Eds.), *Handbook of applied behavior analysis* (pp. 206–225). Guilford.

Bickman, L., Rosof-Williams, J., Salzer, M. S., Summerfelt, W. T., Noser, K., Wilson, S. J., & Karver, M. S. (2000). What information do clinicians value for monitoring adolescent client progress and outcomes? *Professional Psychology: Research and Practice, 31,* 70–74.

Call, N. A., Scheithauer, M. C., & Mevers, J. L. (2017). Functional behavioral assessments. In J. K. Luiselli (Ed.), *Applied behavior analysis advanced guidebook: A manual for professional practice* (pp. 41–71). Academic.

Carr, E. G., Taylor, J. C., & Robison, S. (1991). The effects of sever behavior problems in children on the teaching behavior of adults. *Journal of Applied Behavior Analysis, 24,* 523–535.

Cipani, E. (2018). *Functional behavioral assessment, diagnosis, and treatment: A complete system for education and mental health settings* (3rd ed.). Springer.

Common, E. A., & Lane, K. L. (2017). Social validity assessment. In J. K. Luiselli (Ed.), *Applied behavior analysis advanced guidebook: A manual for professional practice* (pp. 73–92). Academic.

Contreras, B. P., Tate, S. A., Morris, S. L., & Kahng, S. W. (2023). A systematic review of the correspondence between descriptive assessment and functional analysis. *Journal of Applied Behavior Analysis, 56,* 146–165.

Cooper, L. J., Wacker, D. P., Sasso, G. M., Reimers, T. M., & Donn, L. K. (1990). Using parents as therapists to evaluate appropriate behavior of their children: Application to a tertiary diagnostic clinic. *Journal of Applied Behavior Analysis, 23,* 285–296.

Cooper, L. J., Wacker, D. P., Thursby, D., Plagmann, L. A., Harding, J., Millard, T., & Derby, M. (1992). Analysis of the effects of task preferences, task demands, and adult attention on child behavior in outpatient and classroom settings. *Journal of Applied Behavior Analysis, 25,* 823–840.

Cote, C. A., Thompson, R. H., Hanley, G. P., & McKerchar, P. M. (2007). Teacher report and direct assessment of preferences for identifying reinforcers for young children. *Journal of Applied Behavior Analysis, 40,* 157–166.

Durand, V. M., & Crimmins, D. (1992). *The Motivation Assessment Scale.* Monaco & Associates.

Exner, J. E. (1993). *The Rorschach: A comprehensive system* (vol. 1, 3rd ed.). Wiley.

Fantuzzo, J. W., Rohrbeck, C. A., Hightower, A. D., & Work, W. C. (1991). Teachers' use and children's preferences of rewards in elementary school. *Psychology in the Schools, 28,* 175–181.

Favell, J. E., & Cannon, P. R. (1976). Evaluation of entertainment materials for severely retarded persons. *American Journal of Mental Deficiency, 81,* 257–361.

Fisher, W. W., Greer, B. D., Shahan, T. A., & Norris, H. M. (2023). Basic and applied research on extinction bursts. *Journal of Applied Behavior Analysis, 56*, 4–28.

Fisher, W. W., Piazza, C. C., Bowman, L. G., & Amari, A. (1996). Integrating caregiver report with systematic choice assessment to enhance reinforcer identification. *American Journal of Mental Retardation, 101*, 15–25.

Fisher, W., Piazza, C. C., Bowman, L. G., Hagopian, L. P., Owens, J. C., & Slevin, I. (1992). A comparison of two approaches for identifying reinforcers for persons with severe and profound disabilities. *Journal of Applied Behavior Analysis, 25*, 491–498.

Gardner, A. W., Spencer, T. D., Boelter, E. W., DuBard, M., & Jennett, H. K. (2012). A systematic review of brief functional analysis methodology with typically developing children. *Education and Treatment of Children, 35*, 313–332.

Handler, L. (1985). The clinical use of the Draw-A-Person test (DAP). In C. S. Newmark (Ed.), *Major psychological assessment instruments* (pp. 165–216). Allyn & Bacon.

Hanley, G. P. (2012). Functional assessment of problem behavior: Dispelling myths, overcoming implementation obstacles, and developing new lore. *Behavior Analysis in Practice, 5*, 54–72.

Hanley, G. P., Iwata, B. A., Lindberg, J. S., & Conners, J. (2003). Response-restriction analysis: I. Assessment of activity preferences. *Journal of Applied Behavior Analysis, 36*, 47–58.

Hanley, G. P., Iwata, B. A., & McCord, B. E. (2003). Functional analysis of problem behavior: A review. *Journal of Applied Behavior Analysis, 36*, 147–185.

Hanley, G. P., Jin, C. S., Vanselow, N. R., & Hanratty, L. A. (2014). Producing meaningful improvements in problem behavior of children with autism via synthesized analyses and treatments. *Journal of Applied Behavior Analysis, 47*, 16–36.

Hatfield, D. R., & Ogles, B. M. (2004). The use of outcome measures by psychologists in clinical practice. *Professional Psychology: Research and Practice, 35*, 485–491.

Hunsley, J., Lee, C. M., Wood, J. M., & Taylor, W. (2015). Controversial and questionable assessment techniques. In S. O. Lilienfeld, S. J. Lynn, & J. M. Lohr (Eds.) (2nd ed.), *Science and pseudoscience in clinical psychology* (pp. 42–82). Guilford.

Iwata, B. A., & DeLeon, I. (1996). *The functional analysis screening tool.* The Florida Center on Self-Injury, University of Florida.

Iwata, B. A., Dorsey, M. F., Slifer, K. J., Bauman, K. E., & Richman, G. S. (1994). Toward a functional analysis of self-injury. *Journal of Applied Behavior Analysis, 27*, 197–209. (Reprinted from Analysis and Intervention in Developmental Disabilities, 2, 3–20, 1982).

Jessel, J., Hanley, G. P., & Ghaemmaghami, M. (2016). Interview-informed synthesized contingency analyses: Thirty replications and reanalysis. *Journal of Applied Behavior Analysis, 49*, 576–595.

Johnston, J. M., Pennypacker, H. S., & Green, G. (2020). *Strategies and tactics of behavioral research and practice* (4th ed.). Routledge.

Kern, L., Dunlap, G., Clarke, S., & Childs, K. E. (1995). Student-assisted functional assessment interview. *Diagnostique, 19*, 29–39.

Lewis, T., Scott, T., & Sugai, G. (1994). The problem behavior questionnaire: A teacher-based instrument to develop functional hypotheses of problem behavior in general education classrooms. *Diagnostique, 19*, 103–115.

Lilienfeld, S. O., Wood, J. M., & Garb, H. N. (2000). The scientific status of projective techniques. *Psychological Science in the Public Interest, 2*, 27–66.

Mace, F. C. (1994). The significance and future of functional analysis methodologies. *Journal of Applied Behavior Analysis, 27,* 385–392.

Melanson, I. J., & Fahmie, T. A. (2023). Functional analysis of problem behavior: A 40-year review. *Journal of Applied Behavior Analysis, 56,* 262–281.

Mihura, J. L., Jowers, C. E., Dumitrascu, N., Villanueva van den Hurk, A. W., & Keddy, P. J. (2022). The specific uses of the Rorschach in clinical practice: Preliminary results from an international survey. *Rorschachiana, 43,* 25–41.

Miltenberger, R. G. (2016). *Behavior modification: Principles and procedures* (6th ed.). Cengage.

Neef, N. A., & Peterson, S. M. (2007). Functional behavior assessment. In J. O. Cooper, T. E. Heron, & W. L. Heward (Eds.), *Applied behavior analysis* (2nd ed.), pp. 500–524. Pearson.

Northup, J., George, T., Jones, K., Broussard, C., & Vollmer, T. R. (1996). A comparison of reinforcer assessment methods: The utility of verbal and pictorial choice procedures. *Journal of Applied Behavior Analysis, 29,* 201–212.

Northup, J., Wacker, D. P., Berg, W. K., Kelly, L., Sasso, G., & DeRaad, A. (1994). The treatment of severe behavior problems in school settings using a technical assistance model. *Journal of Applied Behavior Analysis, 27,* 33–47.

Northup, J., Wacker, D., Sasso, G., Steege, M., Cigrand, K., Cook, J., & DeRaad, A. (1991). A brief functional analysis of aggressive and alternative behavior in an out-clinic setting. *Journal of Applied Behavior Analysis, 24,* 509–522.

O'Neill, R. E., Horner, R. H., Albin, R. W., Sprague, J. R., Storey, K., & Newton, J. S. (1997). *Functional assessment for problem behavior: A practical handbook* (2nd ed.). Brooks/Cole.

Pace, G. M., Ivancic, M. T., Edwards, G. L., Iwata, B. A., & Page, T. J. (1985). Assessment of stimulus preference and reinforcer value with profoundly retarded individuals. *Journal of Applied Behavior Analysis, 18,* 249–255.

Paclawskyj, T., Matson, J., Rush, K., Smalls, Y., & Vollmer, T. (2000). Questions about behavioral function (QABF): Behavioral checklist for functional assessment of aberrant behavior. *Research in Developmental Disabilities, 21,* 223–229.

Phelps, R., Eisman, E. J., & Kohout, J. (1998). Psychological practice and managed care: Results of the CAPP practitioner survey. *Professional Psychology: Research and Practice, 29,* 31–36.

Roane, H. S., Vollmer, T. R., Ringdahl, J. E., & Marcus, B. A. (1998). Evaluation of a brief stimulus preference assessment. *Journal of Applied Behavior Analysis, 31,* 605–620.

Rolider, A., & Van Houten, R. (1993). The interpersonal treatment model. In R. Van Houten & S. Axelrod (Eds.), *Behavior analysis and treatment* (pp. 127–168). Plenum.

Saini, V., Retzlaff, B., Roane, H. S., & Piazza, C. C. (2021). Identifying and enhancing the effectiveness of positive reinforcement. In W. W. Fisher, C. C. Piazza, & H. S. Roane (Eds.), *Handbook of applied behavior analysis* (2nd ed., pp. 175–192). Guilford.

Sattler, J. M. (2001). *Assessment of children: Cognitive applications* (4th ed.). Author.

Schroeder, C. S., & Smith-Boydston, J. M. (2017). *Assessment and treatment of childhood problems: A clinician's guide* (3rd ed.). Guilford.

Skinner, B. F. (1953). *Science and human behavior.* Free Press.

Solanto, M. V. (2018). Executive function deficits in adults with ADHD. In R. A. Barkley (Ed.), *Attention-deficit hyperactivity disorder: A handbook for diagnosis and treatment* (4th ed., pp. 256–266). Guilford.

Stone, A. A., & Shiffman, S. (1994). Ecological momentary assessment (EMA) in behavioral medicine. *Annals of Behavioral Medicine, 16,* 199–202.

Vlaeyen, J. W. S., Wicksell, R. K., Simons, L. E., Gentili, C., De, T. K., Tate, R. L., Vohra, S., Punja, S., Linton, S. J., Sniehotta, F. F., & Onghena, P. (2020). From Boulder to Stockholm in 70 years: Single case experimental designs in clinical research. *The Psychological Record*, *70*, 659–670.

Wacker, D. P., Schieltz, K. M., & Romani, P. W. (2015). Brief experimental analyses of problem behavior in a pediatric outpatient clinic. In H. S. Roane, J. E. Ringdahl, & T. S. Falcomata (Eds.), *Clinical and organizational applications of applied behavior analysis* (pp. 151–177). Academic.

Wallace, M. D., & Iwata, B. A. (1999). Effects of session duration on functional analysis outcomes. *Journal of Applied Behavior Analysis*, *32*, 175–183.

Wieseler, N. A., Hanson, R. H., Chamberlain, T. P., & Thompson, T. (1985). Functional taxonomy of stereotypic and self-injurious behavior. *Mental Retardation*, *23*, 230–234.

Willcutt, E. G. (2018). Theories of ADHD. In R. A. Barkley (Ed.), *Attention-deficit hyperactivity disorder: A handbook for diagnosis and treatment* (4th ed., pp. 391–404). Guilford.

Wolf, M. M. (1978). Social validity: The case for subjective measurement or how applied behavior analysis is finding its heart. *Journal of Applied Behavior Analysis*, *11*, 203–214.

Prescriptive Behavioral Treatment and Supportive Counseling

4

In primary care behavioral pediatrics, while the child is the client and a participant in the consultation process, the caregiver is the primary direct recipient of services. The caregiver, not the practitioner, is seen as the primary change agent and is given the tools and ongoing support to be successful in that role. Such efforts take many forms including health education, procedural guidance, encouragement, and telehealth-based support between appointments. The behavioral pediatrics literature has traditionally referred to these efforts as prescriptive behavioral treatment and supportive counseling, with referral to other needed services as indicated (Blum & Friman, 2000; Friman, 2005, 2008, 2010, 2021; Friman & Blum, 2002). Each of these is explored in this chapter.

Prescriptive Behavioral Treatment

Changing caregiver behavior is an effective, efficient, durable, and socially valid means of changing child behavior. In nearly all cases, the caregiver is more motivated for change than is the child, and the caregiver typically has far more influence over the child's environment than does the practitioner, so working directly with caregivers tends to be wonderfully productive. Every hour of parent consultation may result in hundreds of hours of changed interactions for the child (Wright, Schaefer, & Solomons, 1979), so compared to traditional behavioral healthcare which typically consists of weekly 45-minute individual talk or play therapy sessions, the child is

DOI: 10.4324/9781003371281-5

effectively immersed in therapy around the clock on a daily basis, and the entire family unit benefits (Kazdin, 2005).

Prescriptive behavioral treatment, simply put, is behavioral treatment prescribed by the practitioner for the caregiver to carry out in day-to-day life. As I often explain to my client families, "To be really helpful, I must train you to do in your home what I would do if I lived there." Therapy resides in the hundreds of daily interactions between child and caregiver. Caregivers may be offered carefully sequenced modular treatment components or packages as well as trained in how to shape behavior generally. An overview of effective behavioral training methods, the behavioral parent training approach, modular treatment, and function-based prevention is offered below.

Basic Teaching and Shaping Repertoire for Caregivers

Caregivers need a basic repertoire of teaching skills (Hanley, 2012) and practitioners of behavioral pediatrics are in a great position to provide it. The teach-back method, guided compliance, and behavioral skills training are useful teaching methods and are discussed below. It should be noted that these methods may also be used by practitioners when training caregivers.

Teach-Back

Perhaps the simplest empirically validated approach to training new skills to others is the *teach-back method*, which involves the trainer verbally explaining specific procedural steps and then asking the trainee to teach back the information in their own words. If the trainee stumbles, the process is repeated. Sleiman, Gravina, and Portillo (2023) demonstrated the application and effectiveness of this method to the training and supervision of RBTs. Teach-back is known to be effective across different settings and populations as well as outcome measures including treatment adherence and patient satisfaction (Sleiman *et al.*, 2023). It is therefore a viable option for use in behavioral pediatrics with caregivers, and by caregivers with their own children.

A downside for this method is that behavioral rehearsal – doing rather than simply saying, as discussed in Chapter 2 – is not an integral component. Thus, other methods such as guided compliance and behavioral skills training may be more appropriate given the circumstances or when teach-back alone has proven insufficient.

Guided Compliance

What is now referred to as *three-step guided compliance* was first described by Horner and Keilitz (1975) and involves issuing a verbal directive (Step 1) and, in the absence of compliance, moving to the issuance of prompts from least to most intrusive (i.e., modeling, which is Step 2, followed by physical prompting, which is Step 3; note that this method of improving behavioral compliance and more are discussed further in Chapter 7). Ndoro and colleagues (2006) found caregiver treatment adherence quite important; they differentiated between integral (issuing the verbal directive and waiting up to 5 seconds before beginning to prompt for compliance), deficient (falling short of that procedurally), and embedded directives (embedding the directive within a play activity, for example, without an explicit description of what is expected; they offered the example of "Let's hop like bunnies to the bathroom" with the preschoolers in their study, p. 82), and found integral and embedded directives to work better than deficient directives in increasing the probability of compliance.

Behavioral Skills Training

Behavioral skills training (BST) is a time-tested stepwise approach to teaching everything from social skills (Dogan *et al.*, 2017) and safe infant sleep environments (Mery *et al.*, 2022) to food allergen avoidance (Quiroz *et al.*, 2023), fire safety (Houvouras & Harvey, 2014), abduction prevention skills (Johnson *et al.*, 2005), and prevention of gun play by children (Miltenberger *et al.*, 2004) to the reduction of injuries in youth soccer (Quintero et al., 2019) and football (Tai & Miltenberger, 2017), and even to playing blackjack (Speelman, Whiting, & Dixon, 2015). The stepwise components are *instructions, modeling, rehearsal,* and *feedback*. Instructions involve clearly and explicitly communicating the specific behaviors or sequence of behaviors expected and the specific circumstances in which the expected behavior should be demonstrated. Modeling involves acting out the behavior so the child may observe and then imitate it. Rehearsal refers to the child's practice of the new behavior within the relevant circumstances (i.e., in the presence of discriminative stimuli), which in turn allows for feedback, or the shaping of the new behavior (Miltenberger, 2016). BST represents a critical skill set for practitioners of behavioral pediatrics. It is through our teaching and coaching effectiveness that caregivers are in turn able to teach and coach their own children, gradually and ultimately without needing us.

Behavioral Parent Training

Development of many of the methods underlying prescriptive behavioral treatment has occurred largely under the labels of *behavioral parent training* (BPT) and, to a lesser extent, *parent management training*, with seminal publications and in-house manuals appearing in the mid-1960s into the 1970s (e.g., Budd, Green, & Baer, 1976; Hanf, 1969, 1970; Hanf & Kling, 1973; Hawkins *et al.*, 1966; Herbert & Baer, 1972; Patterson *et al.*, 1975; Wahler *et al.*, 1965; Wolf, Risley, & Mees, 1963). Reitman and McMahon's (2013) account of the origins of BPT is a highly recommended read which serves both as a literature review and an in memoriam to pioneer Connie Hanf. Empirical support for BPT "greatly surpasses the criteria commonly used to make [the] designation of evidence-based treatment", noted Kazdin (2005), "because of the number of studies and independent replications of outcome effects" (p. 226). A recent meta-analysis (Groenman *et al.*, 2022) found BPT effective in reducing distractibility, hyperactivity, impulsive behavior, oppositional behavior, conduct problems, and general impairment from these problem behaviors for children and adolescents. BPT is most commonly associated with the treatment of oppositional and aggressive behavior (Abikoff & Hechtman, 1996; Forehand & Long, 1988) but it is effective with internalizing problems (Eisen, Engler, & Geyer, 1998; Knox, Albano, & Barlow, 1996; Lebowitz *et al.*, 2014), and for those with histories of abuse (Wolfe *et al.*, 1988) as well. Its effectiveness is also established for integrated primary care settings (Gomez *et al.*, 2014).

This approach involves teaching caregivers the fundamentals of authoritative management practices such as differential attending, effective directive delivery, use of positive and negative consequences, and problem solving. A number of treatment packages have been developed for clinician use (e.g., Barkley, 2013; Chorpita & Weisz, 2009; McMahon & Forehand, 2003; McNeil & Hembree-Kigin, 2010) and all assist caregivers in establishing themselves as reinforcers before endeavoring to establish instructional control. Many clinicians offer client families a hybrid version of these packages, with an example similar to mine shared by Schroeder & Smith-Boydston (2017). BPT is effective whether done with individual families or in a group format (Eyberg, Nelson, & Boggs, 2008). Generalization of treatment effects to untreated settings such as the classroom (McNeil *et al.*, 1991) and maintenance at the five-year (Hood & Eyberg, 2003) and even 14-year mark (Long *et al.*, 1994) have been documented.

Notably, a recent policy statement of the American Academy of Pediatrics (AAP) offering information on this approach acknowledges,

"Nonpharmacologic treatments have more durable effects than medications, with documented effects lasting for years" (AAP, 2020, p. 198) and recommends collaborating and referring across disciplines and specialties to ensure children receive the services they need. The AAP recommends referring young children potentially diagnosable with ADHD for BPT before the diagnosis is made (Wolraich *et al.*, 2019). For those already diagnosed with ADHD and on medication, BPT appears to allow lower dosages to be as effective, and to be superior to cognitive-behavioral therapy which is relatively ineffective for ADHD (Kazdin, 2005; Target & Fonagy, 2005). Much more on BPT is found in Chapter 7.

And as will be covered more in Chapter 11, BPT, and indeed prescriptive behavioral treatment generally, may not be helpful in cases in which caregivers are unwilling or unable to follow through very well with recommended procedures. Such cases involve legally mandated participation, caregiver memory or focus issues, antisocial behavior, substance overuse, marital discord, or social isolation and low social support (Allen & Warzak, 2000; Levensky & O'Donohue, 2006; Stocco & Thompson, 2015; Target & Fonagy, 2005).

Modular Treatment

The effectiveness of prescriptive behavioral treatment may be increased with the use of written protocols for caregivers to take home with them (Cox, Tisdelle, & Culbert, 1988). Such handouts may represent or serve as a component of *modular treatment*. Modularity refers to a particular approach to designing and applying therapeutic protocols involving the explicit outlining of strategies and decision rules (Chorpita, Daleiden, & Weisz, 2005). While related, the concept of modular protocols should not be confused with that of treatment manuals (see Zettle, 2020, for discussion) which tend to be more comprehensive, intended for use with particular clinical diagnoses, and standardized across clinicians. Whereas manualized disorder-specific treatment has been found to be more effective than traditional talk therapy (also referred to as individualized treatment; Kuyken, Padesky, & Dudley, 2009), modular transdiagnostic treatment has been found to be more effective than manualized disorder-specific treatment (Weisz *et al.*, 2012).

Modules, then, are shelf-ready protocols that contain strategies for the provider to use and instructions as to prescribed behavioral treatment for the client or caregiver (or teacher, for that matter) to implement for a given problem or set of problems. The protocols themselves are not the sole treatment but augment didactic and in vivo training along with feedback for caregivers.

Chorpita, Daleiden, and Weisz (2005) provided a template for module development which includes a statement of objectives, a list of needed materials, and prompts for data collection, review of client homework, introduction of new material, assigning new homework, performing a rapport-building activity, and briefing the family, and they note that not all steps are necessarily relevant per appointment. Modular protocols I have developed, alternatively, are in the form of handouts for caregivers which outline prescribed procedures. The format of the former (i.e., Chorpita, Daleiden, & Weisz) appears beneficial for systems and training with an eye to treatment fidelity, whereas the latter may be more appropriate for solo providers with more of an eye to treatment adherence.

Selection of modular protocols is informed by case formulation and treatment planning; protocols are strategically sequenced, which may involve using a pre-developed flowchart, or algorithm (Chorpita, Daleiden, & Weisz, 2005). These protocols represent a starting point in the treatment process, and continuous measurement allows a dialing in of the procedures over time. I have developed a clinical flowchart which serves as a general guide for the initial case formulation and start of therapy; the clinical metafactors covered in Chapters 6 through 9 represent the initial module sequence for many of my clients.

Function-Based Prevention

Primary care behavioral pediatrics is about prevention of problems and amelioration of emerging problems before they become worse. As discussed in Chapter 3, the point of doing functional behavior assessment (FBA) is to know what to teach to the child and what to change about the social and physical environment around the child. Among those functional alternatives we might teach to the child are appropriately manding for attention, help, or a break; tolerating delays or denials of their wishes; and certain friendship skills like sharing, saying thank you, and offering others compliments. That described in the FBA literature represent remedial efforts. But with the primary care population in mind, what if we were to teach these skills *proactively* to children who are not yet demonstrating them, along with other skills like responding to their name and complying with directives? Why wait for problem behavior to occur or a functional behavior assessment to be necessary?

Many of these functional alternatives may be considered life skills; Hanley (2012), for example, proposed such skills to include play skills, compliance with directives, appropriately recruiting and maintaining the attention of others, appropriately escaping and avoiding unpleasant situations, appropriately gaining and maintaining preferred materials, and tolerating delays, denials, and termination of preferred events. The Preschool Life Skills Program (Hanley *et al.*, 2007) was designed to increase appropriate, functionally equivalent social skills while reducing the probability of problem behavior typically developing children within preschool classrooms. Hanley and colleagues proposed 13 target skills within four instructional units (Fahmie & Luczynski, 2018; McKeown, Luczynski, & Lehardy, 2021):

Unit 1: Instruction Following
1. Responding appropriately to name
2. Complying with simple instructions
3. Complying with multistep instructions

Unit 2: Functional Communication
4. Requesting assistance (i.e., "help me please")
5. Requesting attention (i.e., "excuse me")
6. Framed requesting to adults (i.e., "excuse me … may I ___?")
7. Framed requesting to peers (i.e., "excuse me … may I ___?")

Unit 3: Delay Tolerance
8. Tolerating delays imposed by adults (i.e., "okay" and waits patiently for 30s)
9. Tolerating delays imposed by peers (i.e., "okay" and waits patiently for 30s)

Unit 4: Friendship Skills
10. Saying "thank you"
11. Acknowledging or complimenting others
12. Offering or sharing
13. Comforting others in distress

Classwide teaching employing behavioral skills training procedures and skills were each taught to the class by the teacher during morning circle time with opportunities to practice the skills throughout the day. Delay tolerance was facilitated with the instructed mediating response, "When I wait quietly, I get what I want" (see also Toner & Smith, 1977). Studies on the effectiveness of this program with typically developing children and those with developmental disabilities have shown problem behavior to be prevented (Luczynski & Hanley, 2013) as well as reduced while improving social competence (Gunning, Holloway, & Grealish, 2020; see also Beaulieu, Hanley, & Roberson, 2012; Hanley, Fahmie, & Heal, 2014; Luczynski, Hanley, & Rodriguez, 2014; McKeown, Luczynski, & Lehardy, 2021; and Robison, Mann, & Ingvarsson, 2020).

The Preschool Life Skills Program was recently adapted for use in the homes of children with autism spectrum disorder with emerging problem behavior. Called the Balance Program (Ruppel *et al.*, 2021), parents are trained how to initiate trials, prompt desired responses via three-step guided compliance training and fading of prompts, differentially reinforce responding, and employ synthesized reinforcement ultimately on an intermittent schedule, with specific skills in mind: responding to name, manding appropriately, complying with directives, and tolerating denial and delay of wishes. This intervention was found to be effective for all four 3- to 4-year-old children with ASD with emerging problem behavior (e.g., whining, yelling, hitting, throwing) in terms of reducing said behavior and improving social skills and instructional control (Ruppel *et al.*, 2021).

Supportive Counseling

Complementing prescriptive behavioral treatment is supportive counseling for the child and caregivers. The broader specialty of clinical behavior analysis includes science-based models of psychotherapy such as acceptance and commitment therapy (ACT; see a recent meta-analysis by Gloster *et al.*, 2020) which may be employed. Supportive counseling in behavioral pediatrics tends to be relatively brief, however, and offers an opportunity for the behavior analyst *to be human*, to provide encouragement for caregivers needing to just talk through recent hardships or to be a sounding board for a child who doesn't feel socially connected to her peers. The behavior analyst might offer the child social skills instruction or guidance for taming a spike in anxiety before having to speak in class. Child visits to see the clinician also serve as an earned privilege. Caregivers are in attendance for some or all of the session to serve as a catalyst for generalization and maintenance.

Another facet of supportive counseling in behavioral pediatrics is health education, or health promotion, which has a long history within ABA given that physical health is largely a product of operant behavior (Normand, Dallery, & Ong, 2015). Health education by behavior analysts working across subspecialties focuses on everything from tooth brushing (Lattal, 1969) and weight loss (Normand, Dallery, & Ong, 2015) to testicular self-examination (Friman *et al.*, 1986), and many of the presenting concerns covered in this book have an associated physical health dimension. As discussed in the Introduction, behavioral pediatrics involves solving common problems of childhood that are behavioral but with physiological factors, those that are medical with behavioral factors, and those with bidirectional causality (Friman, 2021; Friman & Piazza, 2011). The practitioner serves as an authority on a number of topics pertaining to physical health particularly when the topic is behavior impacting physical health which then impacts subsequent behavior. One need not be a sleep specialist to discuss how to improve bedtime to in turn improve cooperation with the morning routine, for example, nor be a pediatric gastroenterologist to discuss how establishing a regular toileting schedule can lead to less constipation, which in turn leads to fewer encopretic episodes. There are also situations requiring knowledge as to medical considerations, such as asking about the possibility of absence seizures when assessing attention-related problems; parents and teachers can be asked to monitor the child, knowing now what to look for.

Referral

Pediatricians and other primary care providers represent the hub of the wagon wheel, sending patients down the spokes to specialists when needed. Behavioral pediatrics is itself out a little way from the primary care hub; many other providers, including specialty physicians, are further down the spokes. Given the importance of ruling out or addressing medical concerns for a range of referral concerns encountered in behavioral pediatrics, the clinician should actively coordinate with the child's primary care physician when referral to other medical specialties is indicated. For example, a child is referred to you by his pediatrician for treatment of encopresis (covered in Chapter 10). In reviewing the history with the child's caregiver, you find that just before seeing the pediatrician he had moved his bowels but frequently withholds stool, and by the time he reaches you he hasn't produced a bowel movement in four days and is complaining of abdominal pain. You suspect a referral to pediatric gastroenterology may be in order, but you will first consult with the referring pediatrician as to your initial findings, your suspicion of constipation, and to inform that you plan to hold off on behavioral treatment until he is seen medically.

I have maintained a growing list of providers and other consultants and agencies which makes referral navigation rather effortless. Care has been taken to ensure that each individual, agency, and service on the list is familiar with my treatment approach, offers evidence-based services, is highly regarded in the community, and knows collaboration and robust communication are desired and welcomed. This directory includes

- Pediatricians
- Pediatric neurologists
- Pediatric urologists
- Pediatric gastroenterologists
- Pediatric endocrinologists
- Pediatric otolaryngologists
- Pulmonologists
- Sleep specialists and labs
- Child and adolescent psychiatrists
- Psychologists and other therapists
- Behavior analysts offering ASD services
- Pediatric dentists
- Speech therapists
- Occupational therapists
- Physical therapists
- Nutritionists
- Academic tutors
- Social skills groups
- Eating disorders programs
- Crisis stabilization agencies
- Residential treatment facilities
- Child Find and early intervention services
- Educational navigation and advocacy
- Homeschooling groups

Additionally, names and contact information for adult counselors and psychiatrists, executive coaches, collaborative divorce attorneys, educational law attorneys, and substance abuse facilities should also be maintained given that many caregivers could use some direction in times of need. These professionals will in turn likely serve as reliable referral sources.

Key Takeaways from this Chapter

- The caregiver, not the child, is the primary recipient of services in behavioral pediatrics, and these services primarily come in the form of prescriptive behavioral treatment and supportive counseling.

- Prescriptive behavioral treatment refers to behavior change procedures prescribed by the clinician for the caregiver to carry out outside of the consultation session. Caregivers, to be effective in their role, require a basic repertoire of teaching skills and to know what fundamentals to teach, and caregivers are trained in these skills and fundamentals. The teach-back and behavioral skills training methods are useful for such purposes, not only in training caregivers but for caregivers to use these methods with their children. Prescriptive behavioral treatment also relies on decades of research and development of behavioral parent training procedures pertaining to authoritative management. These procedures often are packaged in modular protocol format to facilitate standardization and ease of implementation.
- Function-based prevention represents the proactive teaching of what are considered "life skills" traditionally conceptualized as functional alternatives in the context of functional behavior assessment and functional equivalence training.
- Supportive counseling for the child and caregivers involves health education and efforts to maximize buy-in and treatment adherence. Instruction in social skills or relaxation strategies, as examples, is also offered. Clinicians must also refer out to other professionals as indicated, and maintaining a referral list makes this easier to accomplish.

References

Abikoff, H. B., & Hechtman, L. (1996). Multimodal therapy and stimulants in the treatment of children with attention-deficit hyperactivity disorder. In E. D. Hibbs, P. S. Jensen (Eds.), *Psychosocial treatments for child and adolescent disorders: Empirically based strategies for clinical practice* (pp. 341–369). American Psychological Association.

American Academy of Pediatrics (2020). *Pediatric mental health: A compendium of AAP clinical practice guidelines and policies*. American Academy of Pediatrics.

Allen, K. D., & Warzak, W. J. (2000). The problem of parental noncompliance in clinical behavior analysis: Effective treatment is not enough. *Journal of Applied Behavior Analysis, 33*, 373–391.

Barkley, R. A. (2013). *Defiant children: A clinician's manual for assessment and parent training* (3rd ed.). Guilford.

Beaulieu, L., Hanley, G. P., & Roberson, A. A. (2012). Effects of responding to a name and group call on preschoolers' compliance. *Journal of Applied Behavior Analysis, 45*, 685–707.

Blum, N., & Friman, P. C. (2000). Behavioral pediatrics: The confluence of applied behavior analysis and pediatric medicine. In J. Austin & J. E. Carr (Eds.), *Handbook of applied behavior analysis* (pp. 161–186). Context.

Budd, K. S., Green, D. R., & Baer, D. M. (1976). An analysis of multiple misplaced parental social contingencies. *Journal of Applied Behavior Analysis, 9,* 459–470.

Chorpita, B. F., Daleiden, E. L., & Weisz, J. R. (2005). Modularity in the design and application of therapeutic interventions. *Applied and Preventative Psychology, 11,* 141–156.

Chorpita, B. F., & Weisz, J. R. (2009). *Modular approach to therapy for children with anxiety, depression, trauma, or conduct problems (MATCH-ADTC).* PracticeWise.

Cox, D. J., Tisdelle, D. A., & Culbert, J. P. (1988). Increasing adherence to behavioral homework assignments. *Journal of Behavioral Medicine, 11,* 519–522.

Dogan, R. K., King, M. L., Fischetti, A. T., Lake, C. M., Mathews, T. L., & Warzak, W. J. (2017). *Journal of Applied Behavior Analysis, 50,* 805–818.

Eisen, A. R., Engler, L. B., & Geyer, B. (1998). Parent training for separation anxiety disorder. In. J. M. Briesmeister & C. E. Schaefer (Eds.), *Handbook of parent training: Parents as co-therapists for children's behavior problems* (2nd ed., pp. 205–224). Wiley.

Eyberg, S. M., Nelson, M. M., & Boggs, S. R. (2008). Evidence-based psychosocial treatments for children and adolescents with disruptive behavior. *Journal of Clinical Child and Adolescent Psychology, 37,* 215–237.

Fahmie, T. A., & Luczynski, K. C. (2018). Preschool life skills: Recent advancements and future directions. *Journal of Applied Behavior Analysis, 51,* 183–188.

Forehand, R. L., & Long, N. (1988). Outpatient treatment of the acting out child: Procedures, long term follow-up data, and clinical problems. *Advances in Behavior Research and Therapy, 10,* 129–177.

Friman, P. C. (2005). Behavioral pediatrics. In M. Hersen (Ed.), *Encyclopedia of behavior modification and therapy* (Vol. 2, pp. 731–739). Sage.

Friman, P. C. (2008). Primary care behavioral pediatrics. In M. Hersen & A. M. Gross (Eds.), *Handbook of clinical psychology* (Vol. 2; pp. 728–758). Wiley.

Friman, P. C. (2010). Come on in, the water is fine: Achieving mainstream relevance through integration with primary medical care. *The Behavior Analyst, 33,* 19–36.

Friman, P. C. (2021). Behavioral pediatrics: Integrating applied behavior analysis with pediatric medicine. In W. W. Fisher, C. C. Piazza, & H. S. Roane (Eds.), *Handbook of Applied Behavior Analysis* (2nd ed., pp. 408–426). Guilford.

Friman, P. C., & Blum, N. J. (2002). Primary care behavioral pediatrics. In M. Hersen & W. Sledge (Eds.), *Encyclopedia of psychotherapy* (pp. 379–399). Academic.

Friman, P. C., Finney, J. W., Glasscock, S. G., Weigel, J. W., & Christophersen E. (1986). Testicular self-examination: Validation of a training strategy for early cancer detection. *Journal of Applied Behavior Analysis, 19,* 87–92.

Friman, P. C., & Piazza, C. C. (2011). Behavioral pediatrics: Integrating applied behavior analysis with pediatric medicine. In W. W. Fisher, C. C. Piazza, & H. S. Roane (Eds.), *Handbook of applied behavior analysis* (pp. 433–450). Guilford.

Gloster, A. T., Walder, N., Levin, M. E., Twohig, M. P., & Karekla, M. (2020). The empirical status of acceptance and commitment therapy: A review of meta-analyses. *Journal of Contextual Behavioral Science, 18,* 181–192.

Gomez, D., Bridges, A. J., Andrews III, A. R., Cavell, T. A., Pastrana, F. A., Gregus, S. J., & Ojeda, C. A. (2014). Delivering parent management training in an integrated primary care setting: Description and preliminary outcome data. *Cognitive and Behavioral Practice, 21,* 296–309.

Groenman, A. P., Hornstra, R., Hoekstra, P. J., Steenhuis, L., Aghebati, A., Boyer, B. E., Buitelaar, J. K., Chronis-Tuscano, A., Daley, D., Dehkordian, P., Dvorsky, M., Franke, N., DuPaul, G. J., Gershy, N., Harvey, E., Hennig, T., Herbert, S., Langberg, J., Mautone, J. A., Mikami, A. Y., Pfiffner, L. J., Power, T. J., Reijneveld, S. A., Schramm, S. A., Schweitzer, J. B., Sibley, M. H., Sonuga-Barke, E., Thompson, C., Thompson, M., Webster-Stratton, C., Xie, Y., Luman, M., van der Oord, S., & van den Hoofdakker, B. J. (2022). An individual participant data meta-analysis: Behavioral treatments for children and adolescents with attention-deficit/hyperactivity disorder. *Journal of the American Academy of Child & Adolescent Psychiatry, 61*, 144–158.

Gunning, C., Holloway, J., & Grealish, L. (2020). An evaluation of parents as behavior change agents in the Preschool Life Skills program. *Journal of Applied Behavior Analysis, 53*, 889–917.

Hanf, C. (1969). *A two-stage program for modifying maternal controlling during mother-child (M-C) interaction.* Paper presented at the meeting of the Western Psychological Association, Vancouver, British Columbia, Canada.

Hanf, C. (1970). *Shaping mothers to shape their children's behavior.* Unpublished manuscript, University of Oregon Medical School.

Hanf, C., & Kling, J. (1973). *Facilitating parent-child interaction: A two-stage training model.* Unpublished manuscript, University of Oregon Medical School.

Hanley, G. P. (2012). Functional assessment of problem behavior: Dispelling myths, overcoming implementation obstacles, and developing new lore. *Behavior Analysis in Practice, 5*, 54–72.

Hanley, G. P., Fahmie, T. A., & Heal, N. A. (2014). Evaluation of the preschool life skills program in Head Start classrooms: A systematic replication. *Journal of Applied Behavior Analysis, 47*, 443–448.

Hanley, G. P., Heal, N. A., Tiger, J. H., & Ingvarsson, E. T. (2007). Evaluation of a classwide teaching program for developing preschool life skills. *Journal of Applied Behavior Analysis, 40*, 277–300.

Hawkins, R. P., Peterson, R. F., Schweid, E., & Bijou, S. W. (1966). Behavior therapy in the home: Amelioration of problem parent-child relations with the parent in a therapeutic role. *Journal of Experimental Child Psychology, 4*, 99–107.

Herbert, E. W., & Baer, D. M. (1972). Training parents as behavior modifiers: Self-recording of contingent attention. *Journal of Applied Behavior Analysis, 5*, 139–149.

Hood, K. K., & Eyberg, S. M. (2003). Outcomes of parent-child interaction therapy: Mothers' reports of maintenance three to six years after treatment. *Journal of Clinical Child and Adolescent Psychology, 32*, 419–429.

Horner, R. D., & Keilitz, I. (1975). Training mentally retarded adolescents to brush their teeth. *Journal of Applied Behavior Analysis, 8*, 301–309.

Houvouras, A. J., & Harvey, M. T. (2014). Establishing fire safety skills using behavioral skills training. *Journal of Applied Behavior Analysis, 47*, 420–424.

Johnson, B. M., Miltenberger, R. G., Egemo-Helm, K., Jostad, C. M., Flessner, C., & Gatheridge, B. (2005). Evaluation of behavioral skills training for teaching abduction-prevention skills to young children. *Journal of Applied Behavior Analysis, 38*, 67–78.

Kazdin, A. E. (2005). *Parent management training: Treatment for oppositional, aggressive, and antisocial behavior in children and adolescents.* Oxford.

Knox, L. S., Albano, A. M., & Barlow, D. H. (1996). Parental involvement in the treatment of childhood obsessive-compulsive disorder: A multiple baseline examination incorporating parents. *Behavior Therapy, 27*, 93–115.

Kuyken, W., Padesky, C. A., & Dudley, R. (2009). *Collaborative case conceptualization: Working effectively with clients in cognitive-behavioral therapy.* Guilford.

Lattal, K. A. (1969). Contingency management of toothbrushing behavior in a summer camp for children. *Journal of Applied Behavior Analysis, 2*, 195–198.

Lebowitz, E. R., Omer, H., Hermes, H., & Scahill, L. (2014). Parent training for childhood anxiety disorders: The SPACE program. *Cognitive and Behavioral Practice, 21*, 456–469.

Levensky, E. R., & O'Donohue, W. T. (2006). Patient adherence and nonadherence to treatments. In W. T. O'Donohue & E. R. Levensky (Eds.), *Promoting treatment adherence: A practical handbook for health care providers* (pp. 3–14). Sage.

Long, P., Forehand, R., Wierson, M., & Morgan, A. (1994). Does parent training with young noncompliant children have long-term effects? *Behaviour Research and Therapy, 32*, 101–107.

Luczynski, K. C., & Hanley, G. P. (2013). Prevention of problem behavior by teaching functional communication and self-control skills to preschoolers. *Journal of Applied Behavior Analysis, 46*, 355–368.

Luczynski, K. C., Hanley, G. P., & Rodriguez, N. M. (2014). An evaluation of the generalization and maintenance of functional communication and self-control skills with preschoolers. *Journal of Applied Behavior Analysis, 47*, 246–263.

McKeown, C. A., Luczynski, K. C., & Lehardy, R. K. (2021). Evaluating the generality and social acceptability of early friendship skills. *Journal of Applied Behavior Analysis, 54*, 1341–1368.

McMahon, R. J., & Forehand, R. L. (2003). *Helping the noncompliant child: Family-based treatment for oppositional behavior* (2nd ed.). Guilford.

McNeil, C. B., Eyberg, S., Eisenstadt, T. H., Newcomb, K., & Funderburk, B. (1991). Parent-child interaction therapy with behavior problem children: Generalization of treatment effects to the school setting. *Journal of Clinical Child Psychology, 20*, 140–151.

McNeil, C. B., & Hembree-Kigin, T. L. (2010). *Parent-child interaction therapy* (2nd ed.). Springer.

Mery, J. N., Vladescu, J. C., Day-Watkins, J., Sidener, T. M., Reeve, K. F., & Schnell, L. K. (2022). Training medical students to teach safe infant sleep environments using pyramidal behavioral skills training. *Journal of Applied Behavior Analysis, 55*, 1239–1257.

Miltenberger, R. G. (2016). *Behavior modification: Principles and procedures* (6th ed.). Cengage.

Miltenberger, R. G., Flessner, C., Gatheridge, B., Johnson, B., Satterlund, M., & Egemo, K. (2004). Evaluation of behavioral skills training to prevent gun play in children. *Journal of Applied Behavior Analysis, 37*, 513–516.

Ndoro, V. W., Hanley, G. P., Tiger, J. H., & Heal, N. A. (2006). A descriptive assessment of instruction-based interactions in the preschool classroom. *Journal of Applied Behavior Analysis, 39*, 79–90.

Normand, M. P., Dallery, J., & Ong, T. (2015). Applied behavior analysis for health and fitness. In H. S. Roane, J. E. Ringdahl, & T. S. Falcomata (Eds.), *Clinical and organizational applications of applied behavior analysis* (pp. 555–582). Academic.

Patterson, G. R., Reid, J. B., Jones, R. R., & Conger, R. E. (1975). *A social learning approach to family intervention: Families with aggressive children* (Vol. 1). Castalia.

Quintero, L. M., Moore, J. W., Yeager, M. G., Rowsey, K., Olmi, D. J., Britton-Slater, J., Harper, M. L., & Zezenski, L. E. (2020). Reducing risk of head injury in youth soccer: An extension of behavioral skills training for heading. *Journal of Applied Behavior Analysis, 53*, 237–248.

Quiroz, M. J., Schnell-Peskin, L. K., Kisamore, A. N., Watkins, J. D., & Vladescu, J. C. (2023). Teaching children to identify and avoid food allergens using behavioral skills training. *Journal of Applied Behavior Analysis, 56*, 565–574.

Reitman, D., & McMahon, R. J. (2013). Constance "Connie" Hanf (1917–2002): The mentor and the model. *Cognitive and Behavioral Practice, 20*, 106–116.

Robison, M., Mann, T. B., & Ingvarsson, E. T. (2020). Life skills instruction for children with developmental disabilities. *Journal of Applied Behavior Analysis, 53*, 431–448.

Ruppel, K. W., Hanley, G. P., Landa, R. K., & Rajaraman, A. (2021). An evaluation of "Balance": A home-based, parent-implemented program addressing emerging problem behavior. *Behavior Analysis in Practice, 14*, 324–341.

Schroeder, C. S., & Smith-Boydston, J. M. (2017). *Assessment and treatment of childhood problems: A clinician's guide* (3rd ed.). Guilford.

Sleiman, A. A., Gravina, N. E., & Portillo, D. (2023). An evaluation of the teach-back method for training new skills. *Journal of Applied Behavior Analysis, 56*, 117–130.

Speelman, R. C., Whiting, S. W., & Dixon, M. R. (2015). Using behavioral skills training and video rehearsal to teach blackjack skills. *Journal of Applied Behavior Analysis, 48*, 632–642.

Stocco, C. S., & Thompson, R. H. (2015). Contingency analysis of caregiver behavior: Implications for parent training and future directions. *Journal of Applied Behavior Analysis, 48*, 417–435.

Tai, S. S. M., & Miltenberger, R. G. (2017). Evaluating behavioral skills training to teach safe tackling skills to youth football players. *Journal of Applied Behavior Analysis, 50*, 849–855.

Target, M., & Fonagy, P. (2005). The psychological treatment of child and adolescent psychiatric disorders. In A. Roth, & P. Fonagy (Eds.), *What works for whom? A critical review of psychotherapy research* (2nd ed.). Guilford.

Toner, I. J., & Smith, R. A. (1977). Age and overt verbalization in delay-maintenance behavior in children. *Journal of Experimental Child Psychology, 24*, 123–128.

Wahler, R. G., Winkel, G. H., Peterson, R. F., & Morrison, D. C. (1965). Mothers as behavior therapists for their own children. *Behavior Research and Therapy, 3*, 113–124.

Weisz, J. R., Chorpita, B. F., Palinkas, L. A., Schoenwald, S. K., Miranda, J., Bearman, S. K., Daleiden, E. L., Ugueto, A. M., Ho, A, Martin, J., Gray, J., Alleyne, A., Langer, D. A., Southam-Gerow, M. A., Gibbons, R. D., & Research Network on Youth Mental Health (2012). Testing standard and modular designs for psychotherapy treating depression, anxiety, and conduct problems in youth: A randomized effectiveness trial. *Archives of General Psychiatry, 69*, 274–282.

Wolf, W., Risley, T., & Mees, H. (1963). Application of operant conditioning procedures to the behaviour problems of an autistic child. *Behaviour Research and Therapy, 1*, 305–312.

Wolfe, D. A., Edwards, B., Manion, I., & Koverola, C. (1988). Early intervention for parents at risk of child abuse and neglect: A preliminary intervention. *Journal of Consulting and Clinical Psychology, 56*, 40–47.

Wolraich, M. L., Hagan, J. F., Allan, C., Chan, E., Davison, D., Earls, M., Evans, S. W., Flinn, S. K., Froehlich, T., Frost, J., Holbrook, J. R., Lehmann, C. U., Lessen, H. R., Okechukwu, K., Pierce, K. L., Winner, J. D., Zurhellen, W., & Subcommittee on Children and Adolescents with Attention-Deficit/Hyperactivity Disorder (2019). Clinical practice guideline for the diagnosis, evaluation, and treatment of attention-deficit/hyperactivity disorder in children and adolescents. *Pediatrics, 144,* e20192528. doi: 10.1542/peds.2019-2528

Wright, L., Schaefer, A. B., & Solomons, G. (1979). *Encyclopedia of pediatric psychology.* University Park.

Zettle, R. D. (2020). Treatment manuals, single-subject designs, and evidence-based practice: A clinical behavior analytic perspective. *The Psychological Record, 70,* 649–658.

Case Formulation and Treatment Planning

5

The bridge between initial assessment and treatment planning is case formulation. Also known as case conceptualization, this is "the process of utilizing the abundance of information learned about a client to develop hypotheses about the causal, maintaining, exacerbating, and mitigating variables that directly and indirectly influence clinical problems" (Freeman, 2005, p. 757). Case formulation is an active, collaborative process to synthesize client and caregiver experience, theory, and research, normalize and validate their experiences, promote their engagement, make complex multiproblem presentations more manageable, guide the selection and sequence of interventions, identify client strengths and the most cost-efficient interventions, anticipate and address challenges, help problem-solve ineffective treatment, and enable high-quality supervision and consultation (Kuyken, Padesky, & Dudley, 2009). Behavior-analytic case formulation takes all information into account, including broader historical and current contextual information such as how caregivers and their marital relationship are faring and the child's developmental and medical history (Freeman, 2005). The better your case formulation, the more you truly understand the case.

Clinical Metafactors

Few cases in behavioral pediatrics involve only one concern; most cases involve multiple interacting problems. Rather than making a list of

DOI: 10.4324/9781003371281-6

clinical concerns and then working through that list item by item, however, there may be a more efficient way forward. That is to identify and prioritize certain concerns that are likely occasioning and maintaining other concerns on the list. Without addressing these first, moving through the entire list may take much more time, effort, and expense. Effective, efficient, and durable treatment requires knowing what to treat in what sequence.

An optimal case formulation theoretically offers the luxury of addressing only one behavior or class of behavior to in turn have the greatest overall impact for the client (Bergner, 1998; Sturmey, Ward-Horner, & Doran, 2020). According to Bergner (1998), "the determination of [that one factor] at the heart of the client's difficulties will have the status of an *empirical hypothesis* or *theory*, its adequacy to be determined by how well it fits all of the important empirical facts of the case and how fruitful it proves as a generator of successful therapeutic interventions" (pp. 289–290, italics in the original). The case formulation will likely evolve over the course of treatment as you gain insight. The *analysis* in applied behavior analysis, after all, refers to the insight one gets from continuous measurement as the case progresses.

This book proposes the concept of the *clinical metafactor* as an aid to guiding the strategic sequencing of a series of discrete, modular interventions with efficiency and durability of treatment in mind. Relevant metaphors found in the psychology literature are those of the *linchpin*, referring to "the biggest ripple factor" (Bergner, 1998, p. 290) or a "core state of affairs from which all of the client's difficulties issue" (p. 287), and the *keystone* (e.g., McMahon & Forehand, 2003), referring to the wedge stone at the apex of a rock archway without which the entire structure will collapse. The *central underlying mechanism* is another related concept (Persons, 1989). Research lends support to the strategic sequencing of treatment modules based on the metafactor concept (Kidwell *et al.*, 2019; Nelson *et al.*, 2016), with additional support coming from studies on function-based prevention reviewed in Chapter 4. Among the clinical metafactors are sleep-related problems, behavioral noncompliance with caregiver directives, nonacceptance of caregiver decisions, and weak self-advocacy skills. Most clients encountered in behavioral pediatrics already have a solid repertoire of play and leisure skills but they may lack these other fundamentals. Whether the child is medically ill, getting too much screen time, not eating well or getting enough exercise, or experiencing a disordered home life are important considerations which also likely serve as metafactors.

Treatment Planning

The treatment plan is a written, codified version of your case formulation, detailing for your future self (in the context of a busy caseload) and for others what you see as the problem, the goals for treatment, and the means by which those goals will be realized. The plan need not be overly long; as a general rule, the more printed pages, the less likely the plan will be useful to those implementing it. That is, treatment plans should be succinct and serve as a quick reference during and between appointments for all parties. And in behavioral pediatrics, although the child is the legally identified client, the family in terms of overall conceptualization is best considered the client, so the treatment plan may include goals and intervention for caregivers.

Jongsma and colleagues (2023) propose six steps in the development of treatment plans by behavioral healthcare clinicians: selection of the problem to treat, definition of the problem, development of treatment goals, development of short-term treatment objectives, selection and development of the intervention, and determination of the DSM diagnosis (DSM diagnosis is optional for the behavior analyst practicing behavioral pediatrics; see Chapter 2 for more discussion). With behavior-analytic practice in mind, Johnston, Pennypacker, and Green (2020) additionally recommend that treatment plans include identification of the individuals who will be implementing each component, planned measurement procedures, baseline measurement, generalization and maintenance planning, expected duration of treatment, and criteria for determining whether the objectives are met.

As discussed in a classic paper by Hawkins (1974), goals proposed by caregivers sometimes pertain to the reduction of behavioral excesses, when the more effective route would be to train prosocial functional alternative behaviors; similarly, educators sometimes insist upon targeting the acquisition of certain academic or social skills that are, all things considered, inappropriate or irrelevant. Keeping social validity in mind, the clinician has the responsibility to exercise effective leadership at the treatment planning stage, as in all other stages of consultation, to ensure that which is ultimately agreed upon is likely to be the most effective, efficient, and durable path.

Given that most cases encountered in behavioral pediatrics represent multiproblem cases, those problems identified as targets for intervention should be strategically sequenced balancing metafactor considerations with caregiver priorities. For example, when a child is exhibiting bedtime refusal and a chronic sleep deficit, a 0% behavioral compliance rate, picky eating, and homework refusal, these targets for intervention might best be strategically sequenced as 1) behavioral noncompliance, 2) bedtime refusal and sleep deficit, 3) homework refusal, and 4) picky eating, given that incessant noncompliance renders all other goals virtually unattainable, and with better cooperation we may then improve the bedtime routine and increase the number of hours of sleep the child gets. With both cooperation and sleep improved, we may then more efficiently improve the homework routine, owing to a snowball effect. Picky eating, an important but not priority goal of the caregiver, may then be addressed.

Questions to ask yourself to facilitate case formulation and treatment planning once you have collected information from the history questionnaire, record review, clinical interviews, and observations, may include the following:

• Are there any potential masquerading medical concerns (discussed in Chapter 12)? Picky eaters who are also putting their fingers in their mouths a lot and complaining of leg discomfort at night may require blood work as iron may be low. Acute onset depression in older children may be the result of hypothyroidism. When was the most recent physical and did it include blood work? Is there a family history of low iron or Hashimoto's disease? Are there any reasons to refer this client to a physician prior to starting behavioral treatment?

• Are there any reasons to refer this *caregiver* to services and resources that will predictably improve functioning, treatment adherence, and chances of success with this case?

• How might I strategically sequence the treatment of these target behaviors based on consideration of metafactor status? How do the metafactors of sleep health, behavioral compliance, toleration of denial and delay, and self-advocacy look? More than an hour less sleep than guidelines recommend (see Ferber, 2006, and Chapter 6) may require an initial focus on optimizing sleep health, but if the baseline behavioral compliance rate is under 40%, perhaps noncompliance should first be addressed in order to make sleep treatment more effective.

• What are the predominant concerns and where and with whom are they most observed?

• Are the problems limited to the home setting, or do they occur at school as well? Are there different problems in different settings? At school, is the problem limited to only one teacher, classroom, academic subject, or specific task such as writing?

- Who will be your primary change agent (i.e., the person who will receive the most consultation and training from you)? Who else should be involved in a consultation? If the family employs an au pair, nanny, or frequent babysitters, should they also be trained? How about grandparents who frequently watch the child?

- If you could only offer the family one tip, what tip would likely lead to more success for the family? In the event of anxiety-based concerns, might a discussion of the role of negative reinforcement and avoidance versus exposure be helpful? If there is constant yelling and bickering in the house, might a discussion of differential attending with extinction lead to less arguing?

- How will I operationally define each target behavior and outcome? Does the caregiver agree with these definitions?

- What is our long-term vision for success? How may we quantify this?

- What are specific long-term goals per target behavior across sets of particular circumstances? How may we state these in measurable terms?

- What might the stepping stones, or short-term objectives, be along the path to reaching each long-term goal? How may we state these in measurable terms?

- What science-based treatment packages and procedures are most appropriate for each target behavior?

- How may I establish baseline for each target behavior?

- What measures are most appropriate for each target behavior? Should I use frequency, duration, latency, or rate?

- What criteria can be established to tell us we have met our goals?

- Besides referring caregivers to needed services and resources at the outset of the consultation process, what other steps may I take to program for generalization and maintenance of treatment effects?

- Once underway, do I need to adjust the plan in any way in order to improve effectiveness, efficiency, durability, and acceptability of treatment?

Intervention selection and sequencing are based on all available clinical information, professional literature, and goals and objectives; Chapters 6 through 10 of this book offer guidance for specific clinical problems, and Chapter 11 offers direction as to prediction and facilitation of caregiver treatment adherence which may or may not arise as a clinical problem in its own right to then be included in the treatment plan.

Key Takeaways from this Chapter

- Case formulation, or case conceptualization, is the bridge between initial assessment and treatment planning, representing a synthesis of all information, insights, and likely helpful treatment approaches and methods.
- Clinical metafactors are facets of clinical presentations that likely occasion and maintain other facets; targeting metafactors theoretically should result in a snowball effect as goals are sequentially addressed. Problems such as bedtime refusal and sleep deficit, behavioral noncompliance, poor toleration of denial and delay, and poor self-advocacy skills may be considered metafactors.
- The treatment plan is a tangible result of case formulation efforts and should include operationally defined target behaviors, short- and long-term treatment goals, treatment approaches and procedures selected, names and roles of those who will be implementing prescribed procedures, planned measurement procedures, baseline measurement, generalization and maintenance planning, expected duration of treatment, and criteria for determining when objectives are met.

References

Bergner, R. M. (1998). Characteristics of optimal clinical case formulations: The linchpin concept. *American Journal of Psychotherapy, 52,* 287–300.

Ferber, R. (2006). *Solve your child's sleep problems (rev. ed.).* Fireside.

Freeman, K. A. (2005). Case conceptualization. In M. Hersen, A. M. Gross, & R. S. Drabman (Eds.), *Encyclopedia of behavior modification and cognitive behavior therapy* (vol. 2), pp. 757–761. Sage.

Hawkins, R. P. (1974, March). *Who decided "that" was the problem? Two stages of responsibility for applied behavior analysts.* Paper presented at the Drake Conference on Professional Issues in Behavior Analysis, Des Moines, IA. https://files.eric.ed.gov/fulltext/ED092829.pdf

Johnston, J. M., Pennypacker, H. S., & Green, G. (2020). *Strategies and tactics of behavioral research and practice* (4th ed.). Routledge.

Jongsma, A. E., Peterson, L. M., McInnis, W. P., & Bruce, T. J. (2023). *The child psychotherapy treatment planner* (6th ed.). Wiley.

Kidwell, K. M., McGinnis, J. C., Nguyen, A. V., Arcidiacono, S. J., & Nelson, T. D. (2019). A pilot study examining the effectiveness of brief sleep treatment to improve children's emotional and behavioral functioning. *Children's Health Care, 48,* 314–331.

Kuyken, W., Padesky, C. A., & Dudley, R. (2009). *Collaborative case conceptualization: Working effectively with clients in cognitive-behavioral therapy.* Guilford.

McMahon, R. J., & Forehand, R. L. (2003). *Helping the noncompliant child: Family-based treatment for oppositional behavior* (2nd ed.). Guilford.

Nelson, T. D., Van Dyk, T. R., McGinnis, J. C., Nguyen, A. V., & Long, S. K. (2016). Brief sleep intervention to enhance behavioral parent training for noncompliance: Preliminary findings from a practice-based study. *Clinical Practice in Pediatric Psychology, 4,* 176–187.

Persons, J. (1989). *Cognitive therapy in practice.* Norton.

Sturmey, P., Ward-Horner, J., & Doran, E. (2020). Structural and functional approaches to psychopathology and case formulation. In P. Sturmey (Ed.), *Functional analysis in clinical treatment* (2nd ed.), pp. 1–23. Academic.

Pediatric Sleep Problems **6**

A good majority of children, in my experience, enter outpatient behavioral health services with at least a 90-minute nightly sleep deficit. This observation is corroborated by data showing that most children – up to 70% of neurotypical children and 85% of those with developmental disorders – exhibit problem sleep (Mindell & Owens, 2009; National Sleep Foundation, 2004; Piazza, Fisher, & Kahng, 1996). Children who must be awakened on school days, who tend to sleep in for two or more hours on weekends, and who fall asleep in the car or take naps after school are likely getting insufficient or nonrestorative sleep. A full 69% of children up to age 12 do not fall asleep without an adult present, 42% do not have a consistent bedtime, and 18% consume caffeine on a daily basis (Owens & Jones, 2011). Almost all adolescents live in a relatively constant state of sleep deprivation (Babcock, 2011; Carskadon, 1999; Meltzer & Montgomery-Downs, 2011). Because caregivers may not report concerns about sleep or consider sleep as a factor, and given evidence that improving suboptimal sleep health before addressing many other referral concerns makes overall treatment more effective and efficient (Kidwell *et al.*, 2019; Nelson *et al.*, 2016), sleep is considered an important metafactor.

Despite the tendency for pediatricians to tell parents their children will outgrow sleep problems (Mindell *et al.*, 1994), evidence says otherwise (Johnson *et al.*, 2018). Sleep problems at 8 months of age predict continued sleep problems at age 3 (Zuckerman, Stevenson, & Bailey, 1987). Sleep problems during the preschool years predict persistent sleep problems (Kataria, Swanson, & Trevathan, 1987); anxiety, hyperactivity, and conduct

DOI: 10.4324/9781003371281-7

problems over three years later (Gregory *et al.*, 2004); and anxiety, depression, attention problems, and aggression in adolescence (Gregory & O'Connor, 2002).

Shorter sleep means increased likelihood of shorter stature (Walker, 2017), obesity (Hart, Cairns, & Jelalian, 2011), compromised immune system and more likelihood of catching colds (Cohen *et al.*, 2009), worse vaccine response (Walker, 2017), diabetes (Flint *et al.*, 2007; Javaheri *et al.*, 2011; Schmid, Hallschmid, & Schultes, 2014), hypertension (Walker, 2017) and hypercholesterolemia (Meltzer & Crabtree, 2015) as well as a doubled risk of later cancer and certain types of dementia (Walker, 2017). It results in daytime sleepiness (Liu *et al.*, 2005), lower tested IQ (Gruber *et al.*, 2010), poor academic functioning (Fallone, Owens, & Deane, 2002; Mindell, Owens, & Carskadon, 1999), anxiety (Alfano, Ginsburg, & Kingery, 2007), tantrums (Zuckerman, Stevenson, & Bailey, 1987), and food refusal (Reed *et al.*, 2005). Injuries in general (Koulouglioti, Cole, & Kitzman, 2008; National Sleep Foundation, 2012) and sports injuries (Milewski *et al.*, 2014) are more common with less sleep.

Sleep problems in children affect the environment around them, too, increasing the likelihood of parental depression, anger, stress (Adams & Rickert, 1989; Alfano, Ginsburg, & Kingery, 2007; Mindell & Durand, 1993; Mindell, Kuhn, & Lewin, 2006; Mindell *et al.*, 2009), and divorce (Symon *et al.*, 2005). Parents of these children get less sleep and experience more daytime drowsiness, poor concentration during work hours, worse mood, and drowsy driving (Boergers *et al.*, 2007; Meltzer & Mindell, 2007). Solving child sleep problems improves overall family functioning, including marital satisfaction and parental depression, anger, and perceived stress (Adams & Rickert, 1989; Alfano, Ginsburg, & Kingery, 2007; Mindell & Durand, 1993; Mindell, Kuhn, & Lewin, 2006; Mindell *et al.*, 2009).

There is good reason to see sleep problems as a potential masquerading condition (discussed in more detail in Chapter 12) leading to misdiagnosis. Recall that two of the most common referral concerns for children are anxiety and ADHD. Almost 90% of children with anxiety have sleep problems (Mindell & Owens, 2009), and while anxiety certainly causes challenges with sleep onset and maintenance, inadequate sleep is known to worsen anxiety by among other things increasing reactivity of the amygdala by more than 60% (Walker, 2017). Similarly, sleep problems occur in almost 75% of children diagnosed with ADHD (Noble, O'Laughlin, & Brubaker, 2012), and while the characteristic behaviors summarized as ADHD can certainly impact the bedtime routine, insufficient sleep is known to produce attention problems (Davidson *et al.*, 2022), difficulties with memory and executive functioning (Beebe, Rose, & Amin, 2010; Sadeh, Gruber, & Raviv,

2003), hyperactivity (Knight & Dimitriou, 2019; Mindell & Owens, 2009), more next-day functional avoidance behavior during demand conditions (Kennedy & Meyer, 1996), and poor emotional and behavioral regulation (Davidson *et al.*, 2022; Gruber, Cassoff *et al.*, 2012; Gruber, Michaelsen, *et al.*, 2012). That is, it is assumed that some percentage of children with a diagnosis of ADHD is misdiagnosed (Beebe, 2011; Knight & Dimitriou, 2019; Ribeiro *et al.*, 2015) and this may be partly due to the failure of many diagnosticians to ask about sleep (National Sleep Foundation, 2004).

The literature and range of competencies pertaining to pediatric sleep assessment and treatment are enormous and a comprehensive review would be well beyond the scope of this chapter. The following is intended to enable the reader to address problems commonly encountered in behavioral pediatrics, and to meaningfully collaborate with multidisciplinary professionals. Readers interested in a deeper dive are directed to Meltzer and Crabtree (2015), Perlis, Aloia, and Kuhn (2011), Ferber (2006), Owens and Mindell (2005), and Friman (2005), among other excellent resources.

Assessment of Sleep Health

Assessment methods pertaining to sleep health that may be used by practitioners of behavioral pediatrics include clinical interviews, sleep questionnaires, sleep diaries, and direct behavioral assessments. These are discussed below. Before we get to that, however, it is important to review what healthy sleep looks like.

Sleep Requirements by Age

Ferber's (2006) sleep guidelines encourage eleven hours of sleep per night for 4-year-olds, ten hours for 10-year-olds, and nine hours for 17-year-olds, plus or minus 30 minutes. In the general population, there appears to be about a 90-minute gap between these requirements and what kids typically get beginning in the preschool years and about a two-hour gap by adolescence (Mindell & Owens, 2009). This difference is referred to as a *sleep deficit*, or *sleep debt*. Bedtime scheduling should take age, sleep requirement, and wake-up time into account, plus allowing about 20 minutes to fall asleep (Gellis & Lichstein, 2009). Over 90% of children nap at age 3 but by age 5 only 25% still need a nap (Meltzer & Crabtree, 2015). Outgrowing naps is a sign of brain maturation.

Sleep Stages

We essentially live in three distinct states of awareness: awake, asleep but dreaming, and asleep but not dreaming (Ferber, 2006). The dream state is called REM sleep, which stands for rapid eye movement. During REM sleep, our body is paralyzed with the exception of ocular and respiratory musculature, with some mild twitching of the hands, legs, and face. The brain is active; most of our dreaming, including nightmares, occur during REM sleep. No sweating or shivering occurs during REM, but breathing, heart rate, and blood pressure are irregular. We may be awakened easily during REM and transition to alertness may be rapid (Ferber, 2006). The non-dream state is referred to as non-REM sleep which is subdivided into Stage I (drowsiness, nodding off), Stage II (light sleep, easily awakened), and Stage III (deep sleep, hard to wake). Healthy sleep in children and adults involves sleep cycles approximately 90 minutes in duration throughout the night with more deep sleep at first followed by longer intervals of REM sleep. The first two sleep cycles, usually representing the first three hours of sleep, involve lots of deep sleep, and subsequent cycles are relatively devoid of deep sleep until the final one of the night (provided sufficient sleep scheduling). Beginning with the third cycle, there is a lot of light sleep mixed with REM sleep. We tend to wake momentarily between cycles to instinctively check on our safety (i.e., did anything change in the sleep environment since I fell asleep?), decide if we need to visit the bathroom, and shift sleeping position.

Assessment Methods

Caregiver Interview

Meltzer and Crabtree's (2015) excellent book on pediatric sleep recommends first conducting a thorough clinical interview with caregivers, obtaining the history with regard to typical sleep scheduling and patterns, and screening for sleep disorders (i.e., obstructive sleep apnea, restless legs syndrome, periodic limb movement disorder, narcolepsy, insomnia, delayed sleep phase, parasomnias such as sleepwalking or night terrors, nocturnal enuresis, excessive daytime sleepiness); medical; developmental; behavioral health; family history of sleep disorders and behavioral health challenges; and social and environmental history (e.g., home life, peer socialization, caffeine use, diet, academic performance, access to screen electronic devices near and after lights-out, significant life events, potential disagreement across shared visitation households as to bedtime). Caregivers' goals and expectations should be solicited; as Meltzer and Crabtree note, parents who hope for no crying during sleep training, for example, would benefit more from a modified extinction approach (described below). Interventions not tailored to the needs and expectations of the family may be futile. Caregivers are the primary informants for children up to age 7; children 8 and older tend to know more about their own sleep than their parents (Owens et al., 2000; Paavonen et al., 2000) and should therefore also be interviewed about their sleep.

Sleep problems stem from an interaction among biological, circadian, temperamental, environmental, and behavioral variables (Morgenthaler et al., 2006) involving "predisposing, precipitating, and perpetuating factors" highly influenced by "developmental, environmental, and cultural context" (p. 1278). Functional behavior assessment is valuable in the assessment of problem bedtime and delayed sleep onset (Didden, Sigafoos, & Lancioni, 2011; see also Jin, Hanley, & Beaulieu, 2013; McLay et al., 2019; and McLay et al., 2021). Many important antecedent factors may be considered and queried:

- Is the child being given caffeine or is a prescribed psychostimulant still psychoactive in the evening?
- Is the run-up to bedtime typically hurried, or gradual?
- Is bath time happening too close to bedtime so body temperature is unable to fall in time?
- Is there roughhousing right before bed?
- Are favored books or toys available after lights-out?
- Is sleep onset dependent upon parental presence?
- Is there too much noise in the house after lights-out?
- Is bedtime or the bedtime routine unpredictable from one night to the next?
- Is the bedroom too hot or too cold?
- Is the pillow or mattress uncomfortable?

As to consequences potentially maintaining bedtime problems or delayed sleep onset, does the caregiver sometimes return to the bedroom upon being verbally summoned by the child after lights-out, or reliably interact with the child when leaving the bedroom? As observed by Schnoes (2011), a bedtime routine ending with the child alone in a darkened room is functionally equivalent to time-out (see the next section for more on the time-out concept and procedure), and in this light, it should not surprise us that many children would rather bask in the sunlight of attention than lie awake and bored in a dark room alone. Bedtime refusal and curtain calls (i.e., leaving the room after lights-out) likely reflect historically reinforced extinction bursts.

Practitioners will likely encounter the most sleep-related problems among children of preschool age for a number of reasons. These children have recently moved from their cribs to beds which gives them more opportunity to leave the bed and bedroom. Furthermore, enlarged tonsils and adenoids at this age lead to breathing problems like obstructive sleep apnea, and parasomnias like night terrors and sleepwalking are most common at this age (Meltzer & Crabtree, 2015).

Sleep onset, according to Blampied and France (1993), "can be thought of as the end of an operant chain ... that begins with bed-preparation behaviors and ends in a period of behavioral quietude just before sleep begins" (p. 478). Starting at an even earlier point on the nightly timeline, we might consider the extent to which the child is able to engage in self-quieting by day. Self-quieting may be defined as the child's ability to self-calm when upset (Christophersen & McConahay, 2011). Is the child able to self-quiet within, say, 15 minutes? Or, does the caregiver reliably intervene when the child is upset? If the child is unable to self-calm independently by day, or is not given the opportunity to try, then the child's ability to self-quiet when left alone at bedtime is probably poor. Self-quieting skills, on the other hand, allow the onset of the behavioral quietude mentioned by Blampied and France that is necessary for sleep onset.

Reports of disordered breathing, morning headaches, or limb movements during sleep (or children with sufficient sleep allotment but sleep does not appear restorative) may result in a referral for a sleep study, or Type I polysomnography (PSG), after coordinating with the child's pediatrician. A sleep study represents the medical evaluation of possible underlying factors that disrupt sleep. This is done in a medical setting such as a sleep lab and is considered the gold standard for evaluating sleep-related breathing disorders like obstructive sleep apnea and hypoventilation. It is also used to assess for nocturnal seizures and periodic limb movement disorder (Rundo & Downey, 2019). Type II through IV represent pared-down versions of the PSG that may be done in the home based upon referral concern.

Information on iron intake is important to collect whenever there is evidence of restless legs syndrome (RLS), as low serum ferritin (<50 ng per mL) is a known cause (Durmer & Quraishi, 2011). Picky eaters also are more likely to suffer from RLS given low iron intake from refusal of meats and vegetables. The estimated prevalence of RLS in the pediatric population is 2% but it is seen in up to 44% of those with an ADHD diagnosis.

Sleep Diary

The sleep diary is essentially a one- to two-week baseline collected by caregivers on such things as bedtime refusal, lights-out time, onset latency, frequency and duration of night awakenings, rise time, nap frequency and duration, and any additional information that might be useful (Owens & Mindell, 2011; Meltzer & Crabtree, 2015). Data collection can be continued throughout the initial assessment process as well as treatment.

Sleep Questionnaires

Questionnaires augment the information gained via interviews and sleep diaries. Well-established sleep questionnaires available (Lewandowski, Toliver-Sokol, & Palermo, 2011) include the Brief Infant Sleep Questionnaire (Sadeh, 2004) for birth through 29 months of age, Children's Sleep Habits Questionnaire (Owens, Spirito, & McGuinn, 2000) for ages 4 to 10, Pediatric Sleep Questionnaire (Chervin et al., 2000) for ages 2 to 18, and specifically for use with the autism spectrum disorder population, Sleep Disturbance Scale for Children (Bruni et al., 1996) for ages 5 to 15. Hanley's (2005) Sleep Assessment and Treatment Tool is also an option.

Direct Behavioral Assessment

Direct behavioral assessment (Luiselli, 2021) may include frequency data of calling out and leaving the bedroom (Freeman, 2006), audio recordings of crying and vocal disruption (Moore et al., 2007), and occurrence intervals of sleep and wakefulness (O'Reilly, Lancioni, & Sigafoos, 2004; Piazza & Fisher, 1991). Momentary time sampling is a particularly useful method of data collection for sleep-related measurement as it involves predetermining the recording interval (e.g., 30 minutes) and then observing and recording at the end of each interval (Luiselli et al., 2005). Videosomnography, or video recording during sleep, makes reliable observational measurement possible and practical and may serve as a check on client or caregiver sleep diary reliability (Jin, Hanley, & Beaulieu, 2013; see also van Deurs et al., 2021, and for a more detailed review, Luiselli, 2021).

Another direct measurement method is actigraphy. Paired with the sleep diary, actigraphy involves wearing a watch-like device (Fitbit and Apple watches represent alternatives) on the nondominant wrist to measure movement, and combining the two sources of data to examine sleep onset, duration, and quality. Actigraphy is appropriate in the evaluation of insomnia, circadian rhythm sleep-wake disorders, sleep apnea, and central disorders of hypersomnolence (Smith *et al.*, 2018). The American Academy of Sleep Medicine's sleep parameters (Morgenthaler *et al.*, 2007) supports the use of wrist actigraphy in the diagnosis of delayed sleep phase disorder.

Treatment of Sleep-Related Problems

Behavioral treatments for pediatric sleep problems enjoy strong empirical support. Because treatment varies according to the specifics of the problem, initial assessment is critical. Treatment can involve health education as well as antecedent and consequent manipulation, and a number of science-based treatment procedures have been developed.

Health Education

Perhaps the most common sleep-related intervention is simple psychoeducation about children's sleep needs; in many cases, an earlier bedtime is sufficient. Again, 4-year-olds need about eleven hours of sleep, 10-year-olds need about ten, and 17-year-olds need about nine. Additionally, I routinely tell children with sleep deficits that sleep is a human's way of charging to 100% just as plugging in the tablet or phone is the device's way of charging to 100%, and right now (at the start of treatment) they are only charging themselves to maybe 70% and expecting the charge to last all day. This is usually compelling and effective for children needing a little more structure and motivation.

Caregivers may be offered a primer on normal sleep cycling and sleep associations as a rationale for eliminating caregiver presence at sleep onset. Approximately 90 minutes after sleep onset, the child will rouse slightly at the end of the first sleep cycle. If the sleep environment has significantly changed (i.e., a caregiver who was there before is now gone), the child will awaken more fully with an instinct to reinstate the initial conditions. If, on the other hand, a caregiver is not present at sleep onset, the child will notice no difference in the sleep environment and should fall naturally into the next sleep cycle. Other health education interventions may include guidance for caregivers as to the need for sufficient exercise, maintaining a consistent (i.e., "strict") bedtime, withholding caffeine, removing screen electronics at least one hour before lights-out, refraining from roughhousing right before bedtime, removing access to favored books and toys after lights-out, dimming the lighting scheme, and cooling down the ambient temperature. Medication subscribers should be alerted to sleep issues as well.

Sleep terrors, usually involving sudden blood-curdling screams in the first third of the night, are non-REM, deep sleep phenomena; they do not represent nightmares and so their name reflects their effect on caregivers and siblings, not on the child exhibiting them. The child may be wide-eyed and flailing about during an episode but is nonetheless asleep. Caregivers require guidance to simply maintain the child's safety while not attempting to wake or calm the child during a sleep terror or talking about it later. Children do not recall these episodes and may be embarrassed or frightened if confronted later about them. Sleep terrors, sleep-walking, and other parasomnias are more likely in cases of sleep deficit and poor sleep habits, and may be successfully treated simply by ensuring sufficient and regular sleep.

Unmodified Extinction Approach

Unmodified extinction in the context of bedtime training refers to saying goodnight and then completely ignoring all bids for attention until morning, while monitoring to ensure safety. If the child leaves the bedroom, the caregiver "robotically returns" the child back to bed without eye contact, talking, or tucking him or her back into bed lovingly as before, and this robotic return procedure is repeated as many times as needed until the child remains in bed. This is used for curtain calls immediately after lights-out and in the middle of the night when the child appears at the caregiver's bedside. It can be critical to spend some bonding time with the child before lights-out to demonstrate love and acceptance available by day and announce the after-bedtime policy to facilitate an immediate understanding of the conditions being engineered by the caregiver. The unmodified extinction approach to bedtime training is well supported and designated as a guideline recommendation by the American Academy of Sleep Medicine (Morgenthaler *et al.*, 2006), and tends to work within about three nights given high treatment adherence by caregivers.

This approach is not for all children nor is it for all caregivers, many of whom may convince themselves such procedures are tantamount to abuse and risk damaging the caregiver-child bond. Studies have found this to be false, however (e.g., Price *et al.*, 2012). Nonetheless, a less intensive alternative is the modified extinction approach, below.

Modified Extinction Approach

Whereas the unmodified extinction approach takes about three nights, the modified, or graduated, extinction approach takes about two weeks for success (Meltzer & Crabtree, 2015). Interventions under this approach are categorized in terms of with and without parental presence after lights-out. With parental presence, the caregiver says goodnight and then sits in a chair next to the bed without talking and leaves the room once the child is asleep. Each night the chair gets progressively closer to the doorway, ultimately being placed outside the doorway so only the caregiver's foot is visible to the child. Without parental presence, the caregiver says goodnight and then essentially switches from checking on the child contingent upon the child calling out, to noncontingent, which is now on the caregiver's schedule and insensitive to the child's calling out. Checking on the child is frequent at first and less frequent over time. Either way, in the event the child leaves the room in the middle of the night, he or she is robotically returned to the room with no talking or eye contact, and repeated as necessary.

Flashlight Treasure Hunts

For children who are afraid of the dark, a toy may be hidden in the bedroom just before bedtime each night; children are given a flashlight and enter their darkened room to hunt for the hidden toy. The toy may be big and easy to find at first, and night after night smaller and harder to find. Locating the toy earns them a big hug and congratulations (Meltzer & Crabtree, 2015). This intervention is geared to desensitize the child to the sleep environment, associating it with fun rather than fright. More intervention options exist for addressing fear of the dark or being alone at night; see the anxiety section of Chapter 10 for more.

Daytime Training of Self-Quieting Skills

Children who struggle to self-quiet after lights-out tend to similarly struggle by day and typically require or expect correction or soothing from a caregiver. Christophersen and McConahay (2011; see also Blum & Friman, 2000) recommend shaping self-quieting during the day to help the child settle in at lights-out; this intervention may be more palatable for caregivers who struggle to adhere to extinction procedures (i.e., ignoring). Children can learn this skill but they must be given the opportunity to do so. Christophersen and McConahay suggest establishing a period of time-in (see Chapter 7 for more) during which there are no warnings or threats, and when the child engages in, for example, interrupting of the adults, the caregiver may simply say "stop interrupting" followed by complete ignoring (i.e., no correction, no answering of any kind, and no eye contact) until appropriate behavior and a respectful countenance have returned. The child must be able to see that the caregiver is not upset. When the child has self-quieted, time-in resumes.

Bedtime Fading

When an earlier bedtime must be established, but the child is not sleepy at that hour, bedtime fading may be used. The caregiver maintains a sleep diary for at least a week to establish when the child typically falls asleep. The child's new bedtime is set for 30 to 45 minutes before typical sleep onset; after about a week when sleep onset latency has fallen below 30 minutes, bedtime is set for 15 minutes earlier than that. Bedtime is then adjusted by 15 minutes more each subsequent week or so until reaching a target bedtime consistent with sleep requirement guidelines (Meltzer & Crabtree, 2015). Weekends should be treated no differently than weeknights: no later bedtimes, and no sleeping in.

The Sleep Check

An intervention developed in my clinic to help with bedtime is the Sleep Check. This involves the caregiver telling the child at lights-out that he or she will handle a chore or two and then tiptoe in to check whether the child is asleep, and if the child is asleep at the sleep check, he or she will earn a treat or privilege in the morning. This intervention occasions and incentivizes behavioral quietude from pretending to be asleep which is necessary to easily fall asleep. A variation lending empirical support is the Sleep Fairy intervention (Burke, Kuhn, & Peterson, 2004; see also *The Sleep Fairy* storybook by Peterson & Peterson, 2014) that functions like the traditional Tooth Fairy bit.

When the child goes to bed without a fuss and falls asleep quickly, he or she awakens in the morning to find a treat or token under the pillow. The Sleep Fairy visits nightly for a couple of weeks and then intermittently because she has lots of houses to visit (Meltzer & Crabtree, 2015).

The Bedtime Pass

The Bedtime Pass intervention (Friman *et al.*, 1999) helps address challenging bedtime routines and curtain calls. The child is offered a token at bedtime that may be redeemed before onset of sleep for a minute of the caregiver's time to supportively handle an easily satisfied request (e.g., another hug or sip of water). If redeemed after lights-out, the token is returned to the child the next evening at bedtime. If, however, the child does not redeem it after lights-out, it may be redeemed in the morning for a special treat or privilege (Schnoes, 2011), including the ability to stay up 10 minutes later with the caregiver before lights-out. If the child leaves the bed and refuses to give up the pass or leaves the bed again after having redeemed it, the child is matter-of-factly physically ushered back to bed with no discussion. This intervention has been shown to reliably reduce or eliminate bedtime challenges (Freeman, 2006; Friman *et al.*, 1999; Moore *et al.*, 2007).

The Good Morning Light

The Good Morning Light intervention essentially offers the child who cannot yet read a clock a visual cue that it is okay to get out of bed (Meltzer, 2010; Meltzer & Crabtree, 2015). A lamp is placed on a timer to turn off at bedtime and on at wake time. There are now a number of commercial products found under the keyword phrases of "kids alarm clock" or "okay to wake" that serve the same purpose. The child must be told what the light means followed by caregiver enforcement of the rule. A reward component may be paired with this intervention as needed for more effectiveness (Meltzer, 2010).

Key Takeaways from this Chapter

- Sleep-related problems are common in childhood, can have a significant detrimental impact on the child's biological health and daily functioning as well as family dynamics, and tend to continue without treatment.

Unidentified and untreated sleep problems can contribute to misdiagnosis in behavioral health. For these reasons and more, sleep problems are considered a clinical metafactor to be prioritized for treatment.

- Children generally require about eleven hours of sleep per night at age 4, ten hours at age 10, and nine hours at age 17, but they typically get around two hours fewer than that per night.
- Assessment of sleep health involves a combination of clinical interview, use of a sleep diary, sleep questionnaires, and direct assessment which might involve the use of audio or video recording and actigraphy. Functional behavior assessment is a useful assessment component for sleep problems as well. Children may be referred to a sleep lab for a sleep study, also known as polysomnography, when there is suspicion of disordered breathing, morning headaches, or limb movements while sleeping.
- Behavioral treatment of sleep problems enjoys strong empirical support and generally involves some combination of health education, exposure, unmodified or modified extinction, bedtime fading, contingency management, and establishment of stimulus control.

References

Adams, L. A., & Rickert, V. I. (1989). Reducing bedtime tantrums: Comparison between positive routines and graduated extinction. *Pediatrics, 84,* 756–761.

Alfano, C. A., Ginsburg, G. S., & Kingery, J. N. (2007). Sleep-related problems among children and adolescents with anxiety disorders. *Journal of the American Academy of Child and Adolescent Psychiatry, 46,* 224–232.

Babcock, D. A. (2011). Evaluating sleep and sleep disorders in the pediatric primary care setting. *Pediatric Clinics of North America, 58,* 543–554.

Beebe, D. W. (2011). Cognitive, behavioral, and functional consequences of inadequate sleep in children and adolescents. *Pediatric Clinics of North America, 58,* 649–665.

Beebe, D. W., Rose, D., & Amin, R. (2010). Attention, learning, and arousal of experimentally sleep-restricted adolescents in a simulated classroom. *Journal of Adolescent Health, 47,* 523–525.

Blampied, N. M., & France, K. G. (1993). A behavioral model of infant sleep disturbance. *Journal of Applied Behavior Analysis, 26,* 477–492.

Blum, N., & Friman, P. C. (2000). Behavioral pediatrics: The confluence of applied behavior analysis and pediatric medicine. In J. Austin, & J. E. Carr (Eds.), *Handbook of applied behavior analysis* (pp. 161–186). Context.

Boergers, J., Hart, C., Owens, J. A., Streisand, R., & Spirito, A. (2007). Child sleep disorders: Associations with parental sleep duration and daytime sleepiness. *Journal of Family Psychology, 21,* 88–94.

Bruni, O., Ottaviano, S., Giudetti, V., Romoli, M., Innocenzi, M., Cortesi, F., & Giannotti, R. (1996). The Sleep Disturbance Scale for Children (SDSC): Construction and validation of an instrument to evaluate sleep disturbances in childhood and adolescence. *Journal of Sleep Research, 5*, 251–261.

Burke, R. V., Kuhn, B. R., & Peterson, J. L. (2004). Brief report: A "story-book" ending to children's bedtime problems – The use of a rewarding social story to reduce bedtime resistance and frequent night waking. *Journal of Pediatric Psychology, 29*, 389–396.

Carskadon, M. A. (1999). When worlds collide: Adolescent need for sleep versus societal demands. *Phi Delta Kappan, 80*, 348–353.

Chervin, R. D., Hedger, K., Dillon, J. E., & Pituch, K. J. (2000). Pediatric Sleep Questionnaire (PSQ): Validity and reliability of scales for sleep-disordered breathing, snoring, sleepiness, and behavioral problems. *Sleep Medicine Reviews, 1*, 21–32.

Christophersen, E. R., & McConahay, K. H. (2011). Day correction of pediatric bedtime problems. In M. Perlis, M. Aloia, & B. Kuhn (Eds.), *Behavioral treatments for sleep disorders: A comprehensive primer of behavioral sleep medicine interventions* (pp. 311–317). Academic.

Cohen, S., Doyle, W. J., Alper, C. M., Janicki-Deverts, D., & Turner, R. B. (2009). Sleep habits and susceptibility to the common cold. *Archives of Internal Medicine, 169*, 62–67.

Davidson, F., Rigney, G., Brine, S., Speth, T., Miller, L., Rusak, B., Chambers, C., Rajda, M., Begum, E. A., & Corkum, P. (2022). Even a mild sleep restriction can impact daytime functioning in children with ADHD and their typically developing peers. *Behavioral Sleep Medicine, 20*, 21–36.

Didden, R., Sigafoos, J., & Lancioni, G. E. (2011). Unmodified extinction for childhood sleep disturbance. In M. Perlis, M. Aloia, & B. Kuhn (Eds.), *Behavioral treatments for sleep disorders: A comprehensive primer of behavioral sleep medicine interventions* (pp. 257–263). Academic.

Durmer, J. S., & Quraishi, G. H. (2011). Restless legs syndrome, periodic leg movements, and periodic limb movement disorder in children. *Pediatric Clinics of North America, 58*, 591–620.

Fallone, G., Owens, J. A., & Deane, J. (2002). Sleepiness in children and adolescents: Clinical implications. *Sleep Medicine Reviews, 6*, 287–306.

Ferber, R. (2006). *Solve your child's sleep problems (rev. ed.).* Fireside.

Flint, J., Kothare, S. V., Zihlif, M., Suarez, E., Adams, R., Legido, A., & DeLuca, F. (2007). Association between inadequate sleep and insulin resistance in obese children. *The Journal of Pediatrics, 150*, 364–369.

Freeman, K. A. (2006). Treating bedtime resistance with the bedtime pass: A systematic replication and component analysis with 3-year-olds. *Journal of Applied Behavior Analysis, 39*, 423–428.

Friman, P. C. (2005). *Good night, sweet dreams, I love you, now get into bed and go to sleep! How tired parents can solve their children's bedtime problems.* Boys Town.

Friman, P. C., Hoff, K. E., Schnoes, C., Freeman, K., Woods, D. W., & Blum, N. (1999). The Bedtime Pass: An approach to bedtime crying and leaving the room. *Archives of Pediatrics and Adolescent Medicine, 153*, 1027–1029.

Gellis, L. A., & Lichstein, K. L. (2009). Sleep hygiene practices of good and poor sleepers in the United States: An internet-based study. *Behavior Therapy, 40*, 1–9.

Gregory, A. M., Eley, T. C., O'Connor, T. G., & Plomin, R. (2004). Etiologies of associations between childhood sleep and behavioral problems in a large twin sample. *Journal of the American Academy of Child and Adolescent Psychiatry, 43*, 744–751.

Gregory, A. M., & O'Connor, T. G. (2002). Sleep problems in childhood: A longitudinal study of developmental change and association with behavioral problems. *Journal of the American Academy of Child and Adolescent Psychiatry, 41,* 964–971.

Gruber, R., Cassoff, J., Frenette, S., Wiebe, S., & Carrier, J. (2012). Impact of sleep extension and restriction on children's emotional lability and impulsivity. *Pediatrics, 130,* e1155–e1161. 10.1542/peds.2012-0564

Gruber, R., Laviolette, R., Deluca, P., Monson, E., Cornish, K., & Carrier, J. (2010). Short sleep duration is associated with poor performance on IQ measures in healthy school-age children. *Sleep Medicine, 11,* 289–294.

Gruber, R., Michaelsen, S., Bergmame, L., Frenette, S., Bruni, O., Fontil, L., & Carrier, J. (2012). Short sleep duration is associated with teacher-reported inattention and cognitive problems in healthy school-aged children. *Nature and Science of Sleep, 4,* 33–40.

Hanley, G. P. (2005). Sleep Assessment and Treatment Tool [measurement instrument]. Retrieved from practicalfunctionalassessment.files.wordpress.com/2015/06/satt.pdf.

Hart, C. N., Cairns, A., & Jelalian, E. (2011). Sleep and obesity in children and adolescents. *Pediatric Clinics of North America, 58,* 715–733.

Javaheri, S., Storfer-Isser, A., Rosen, C. L., & Redline, S. (2011). Association of short and long sleep durations with insulin sensitivity in adolescents. *The Journal of Pediatrics, 158,* 617–623.

Jin, C. S., Hanley, G. P., & Beaulieu, L. (2013). An individualized and comprehensive approach to treating sleep problems in young children. *Journal of Applied Behavior Analysis, 46,* 161–180.

Johnson, C. R., Smith, T., DeMand, A., Lecavalier, L., Evans, V., Gurka, M., Swiezy, N., Bearss, K., & Scahill, L. (2018). Exploring sleep quality of young children with autism spectrum disorder and disruptive behaviors. *Sleep Medicine, 44,* 61–66.

Kataria, S., Swanson, M. S., & Trevathan, G. E. (1987). Persistence of sleep disturbances in preschool children. *The Journal of Pediatrics, 110,* 642–646.

Kennedy, C. H., & Meyer, K. A. (1996). Sleep deprivation, allergy symptoms, and negatively reinforced problem behavior. *Journal of Applied Behavior Analysis, 29,* 133–135.

Kidwell, K. M., McGinnis, J. C., Nguyen, A. V., Arcidiacono, S. J., & Nelson, T. D. (2019). A pilot study examining the effectiveness of brief sleep treatment to improve children's emotional and behavioral functioning. *Children's Health Care, 48,* 314–331.

Knight, F. L. C., & Dimitriou, D. (2019). Poor sleep has negative implications for children with and without ADHD, but in different ways. *Behavioral Sleep Medicine, 17,* 423–436.

Koulouglioti, C., Cole, R., & Kitzman, H. (2008). Inadequate sleep and unintentional injuries in young children. *Public Health Nursing, 25,* 106–114.

Lewandowski, A. S., Toliver-Sokol, M., & Palermo, T. M. (2011). Evidence-based review of subjective pediatric sleep measures. *Journal of Pediatric Psychology, 36,* 780–793.

Liu, X., Liu, L., Owens, J. A., & Kaplan, D. L. (2005). Sleep patterns and sleep problems among school children in the United States and China. *Pediatrics, 115,* 241–249.

Luiselli, J. K. (2021). Applied behavior analysis measurement, assessment, and treatment of sleep and sleep-related problems. *Journal of Applied Behavior Analysis, 54,* 654–667.

Luiselli, J. K., Magee, C., Sperry, J. M., & Parker, S. (2005). Descriptive assessment of sleep patterns among community-living adults with mental retardation. *Mental Retardation, 43,* 416–420.

McLay, L., France, K., Blampied, N., van Deurs, J., Hunter, J., Knight, J., Hastie, B., Carnett, A., Woodford, E., Gibbs, R., & Lang, R. (2021). Function-based behavioral interventions for sleep problems in children and adolescents with autism: Summary of 41 clinical cases. *Journal of Autism and Developmental Disorders, 51*, 418–432.

McLay, L. K., France, K. G., Knight, J., Blampied, N. M., & Hastie, B. (2019). The effectiveness of function-based interventions to treat sleep problems, including unwanted co-sleeping, in children with autism. *Behavioral Interventions, 34*, 30–51.

Meltzer, L. J. (2010). Clinical management of behavioral insomnia of childhood: Treatment of bedtime problems and night wakings in young children. *Behavioral Sleep Medicine, 8*, 172–189.

Meltzer, L., & Crabtree, V. (2015). *Pediatric sleep problems: A clinician's guide to behavioral interventions*. American Psychological Association.

Meltzer, L. J., & Mindell, J. A. (2007). Relationship between child sleep disturbances and maternal sleep, mood, and parenting stress: A pilot study. *Journal of Family Psychology, 21*, 67–73.

Meltzer, L. J., & Montgomery-Downs, H. E. (2011). Sleep in the family. *Pediatric Clinics of North America, 58*, 765–774.

Milewski, M. D., Skaggs, D. L., Bishop, G. A., Pace, J. L., Ibrahim, D. A., Wren, T. A. L., & Barzdukas, A. (2014). Chronic lack of sleep is associated with increased sports injuries in adolescent athletes. *Journal of Pediatric Orthopaedics, 34*, 129–133.

Mindell, J. A., & Durand, V. M. (1993). Treatment of childhood sleep disorders: Generalization across disorders and effects on family members. *Journal of Pediatric Psychology, 18*, 731–750.

Mindell, J. A., Kuhn, B. R., & Lewin, D. S. (2006). Behavioral treatment of bedtime problems and night wakings in infants and young children. *Sleep, 29*, 1263–1276.

Mindell, J. A., Moline, M. L., Zendell, S. M., Brown, L. W., & Fry, J. M. (1994). Pediatricians and sleep disorders: Training and practice. *Pediatrics, 94*, 194–200.

Mindell, J. A., & Owens, J. A. (2009). *A clinical guide to pediatric sleep: Diagnosis and management of sleep problems* (2nd ed.). Lippincott.

Mindell, J. A., Owens, J. A., & Carskadon, M. A. (1999). Developmental features of sleep. *Child and Adolescent Psychiatric Clinics of North America, 8*, 695–725.

Mindell, J. A., Telofski, L., Weigand, B., & Kurtz, E. S. (2009). A nightly bedtime routine: Impact on sleep in young children and maternal mood. *Sleep, 32*, 599–606.

Moore, B. A., Friman, P. C., Fruzzetti, A. E., & MacAleese, K. (2007). Brief report: Evaluating the bedtime pass program for child resistance to bedtime – A randomized, controlled trial. *Journal of Pediatric Psychology, 32*, 283–287.

Morgenthaler, T. I., Lee-Chiong, T., Alessi, C., Friedman, L., Aurora, R. N., Boehlecke, B., Brown, T., Chesson, A. L., Kapur, V., Maganti, R., Owens, J., Pancer, J., Swick, T. J., & Zak, R. (2007). Practice parameters for the clinical evaluation and treatment of circadian rhythm sleep disorders. An American Academy of Sleep Medicine report. *Sleep, 30*, 1445–1459.

Morgenthaler, T. I., Owens, J., Alessi, C., Boehlecke, B., Brown, T. M., Coleman, J., Friedman, L., Kapur, V. K., Lee-Chiong, T., Pancer, J., & Swick, T. J. (2006). Practice parameters for behavioral treatment of bedtime problems and night wakings in infants and young children: An American Academy of Sleep Medicine report. *Sleep, 29*, 1277–1281.

National Sleep Foundation (2004). *Sleep in America poll*. National Sleep Foundation.

National Sleep Foundation (2012). *Adolescent sleep needs and patterns: Research report and resource guide.* National Sleep Foundation.

Nelson, T. D., Van Dyk, T. R., McGinnis, J. C., Nguyen, A. V., & Long, S. K. (2016). Brief sleep intervention to enhance behavioral parent training for noncompliance: Preliminary findings from a practice-based study. *Clinical Practice in Pediatric Psychology, 4,* 176–187.

Noble, G. S., O'Laughlin, L., & Brubaker, B. (2012). Attention deficit hyperactivity disorder and sleep disturbances: Consideration of parental influence. *Behavioral Sleep Medicine, 10,* 41–53.

O'Reilly, M. F., Lancioni, G. E., & Sigafoos, J. (2004). Using paired-choice assessment to identify variables maintaining sleep problems in a child with severe disabilities. *Journal of Applied Behavior Analysis, 37,* 209–212.

Owens, J. A., & Jones, C. (2011). Parental knowledge of healthy sleep in young children: Results of a primary care survey. *Journal of Developmental and Behavioral Pediatrics, 32,* 447–453.

Owens, J. A., & Mindell, J. A. (2005). *Take charge of your child's sleep: The all-in-one resource for solving sleep problems in kids and teens.* Marlowe.

Owens, J. A., & Mindell, J. A. (2011). Pediatric insomnia. *Pediatric Clinics of North America, 58,* 555–569.

Owens, J. A., Spirito, A., & McGuinn, M. (2000). The Children's Sleep Habits Questionnaire (CSHQ): Psychometric properties of survey instrument for school-aged children. *Sleep, 23,* 1043–1051.

Owens, J. A., Spirito, A., McGuinn, M., & Nobile, C. (2000). Sleep habits and sleep disturbance in elementary school-aged children. *Journal of Developmental and Behavioral Pediatrics, 21,* 27–36.

Paavonen, E. J., Aronen, E. T., Moilanen, I., Piha, J., Rasanen, E., Tamminen, T., & Almqvist, F. (2000). Sleep problems of school-aged children: A complementary view. *Acta Paediatrica, 89,* 223–228. DOI: 10.1080/080352500750028870

Perlis, M., Aloia, M., & Kuhn, B. (2011). *Behavioral treatments for sleep disorders: A comprehensive primer of behavioral sleep medicine interventions.* Academic.

Peterson, J., & Peterson, M. (2014). *The sleep fairy.* Behave'n Kids.

Piazza, C. C., & Fisher, W. (1991). A faded bedtime with response cost protocol for treatment of multiple sleep problems in children. *Journal of Applied Behavior Analysis, 24,* 129–140.

Piazza, C. C., Fisher, W. W., & Kahng, S. W. (1996). A descriptive study of sleep patterns in children with mental retardation and severe behavior disorders. *Developmental Medicine and Child Neurology, 38,* 335–344.

Price, A. M., Wake, M., Ukoumunne, O. C., & Hiscock, H. (2012). Five-year follow-up of harms and benefits of behavioral infant sleep intervention: Randomized trial. *Pediatrics, 130,* 643–651.

Reed, G. K., Dolezal, D. N., Cooper-Brown, L. J., & Wacker, D. P. (2005). The effects of sleep disruption on the treatment if a feeding disorder. *Journal of Applied Behavior Analysis, 38,* 243–245.

Ribeiro, A., Liddon, C. J., Gadaire, D. M., & Kelley, M. E. (2015). Sleep, elimination, and noncompliance in children. In H. S. Roane, J. E. Ringdahl, & T. S. Falcomata (Eds.),

Clinical and organizational applications of applied behavior analysis (pp. 247–272). Academic.

Rundo, J. V., & Downey, R. III. (2019). Polysomnography. *Handbook of Clinical Neurology, 160*, 381–392.

Sadeh, A. (2004). A brief screening questionnaire for infant sleep problems: Validation and findings for an internet sample. *Pediatrics, 113*, e570–e577.

Sadeh, A., Gruber, R., & Raviv, A. (2003). The effects of sleep restriction and extension on school-age children: What a difference an hour makes. *Child Development, 74*, 444–455.

Schmid, S. M., Hallschmid, M., & Schultes, B. (2014). The metabolic burden of sleep loss. *Lancet Diabetes and Endocrinology, 2*, e12.

Schnoes, C. J. (2011). The bedtime pass. In M. Perlis, M. Aloia, & B. Kuhn (Eds.), *Behavioral treatments for sleep disorders: A comprehensive primer of behavioral sleep medicine interventions* (pp. 293–298). Academic.

Smith, M. T., McCrae, C. S., Cheung, J., Martin, J. L., Harrod, C. G., Heald, J. L., & Carden, K. A. (2018). Use of actigraphy for the evaluation of sleep disorders and circadian rhythm sleep-wake disorders: An American Academy of Sleep Medicine systematic review, meta-analysis, and GRADE assessment. *Journal of Clinical Sleep Medicine, 14*, 1209–1230.

Symon, B. G., Marley, J. E., Martin, A. J., & Norman, E. R. (2005). Effect of a consultation teaching behaviour modification on sleep performance in infants: A randomized controlled trial. *The Medical Journal of Australia, 182*, 215–218.

van Deurs, J. R., McLay, L. K., France, K. G., & Blampied, N. M. (2021). Sequential implementation of functional behavior assessment-informed treatment components for sleep disturbance in autism: A case study. *Behavioral Sleep Medicine, 19*, 333–351.

Walker, M. (2017). *Why we sleep: Unlocking the power of sleep and dreams.* Scribner.

Zuckerman, B., Stevenson, J., & Bailey, V. (1987). Sleep problems in early childhood: Continuities, predictive factors, and behavioural correlates. *Pediatrics, 80*, 664–671.

Behavioral Noncompliance

7

Behavioral noncompliance, generally defined as failure to initiate within ten seconds the follow-through of a directive issued by a caregiver or other legitimate authority figure, is one of the most common problem behaviors of childhood (Achenbach & Edelbrock, 1981) and historically one of the most common reasons for referral to outpatient behavioral healthcare (Charlop *et al.*, 1987). Noncompliance represents a clinical metafactor because it predicts mental health diagnosis (Keenan *et al.*, 1998) and the development of many other problem behaviors (McMahon & Forehand, 2003) which impede social, academic, and other important areas of functioning (Kalb & Loeber, 2003; Martens & Kelly, 1993). It is also a predictor of caregiver nonadherence with treatment recommendations; the worse the child's cooperation with the caregiver, the worse the caregiver's cooperation with the clinician (Watson, Foster, & Friman, 2006).

Following the directives and rules of caregivers may be considered a life skill, and improved compliance has been shown to result in decreased subsequent problem behavior (Hanley *et al.*, 2007; Parrish *et al.*, 1986). As observed by Friman (2008), "Success in most life situations requires a reasonable amount of instructional control, yet many children resist following important adult instructions" (p. 728). A child who is relatively compliant with caregiver directives is a coachable one who may thus contact reinforcement without the trial and error of stepwise, contingency-shaped learning (Nergaard & Couto, 2021; Skinner, 1953), potentially benefiting from the previous mistakes of others without having to make those same mistakes.

DOI: 10.4324/9781003371281-8

Typical Compliance Rates

Forehand (1977) reported compliance rates ranging from 60 to 80% for neurotypical preschoolers. Forehand, Gardner, and Roberts (1978) found that children aged 3 to 6 complied 51% of the time but cautioned that their caregivers thwarted their children's success 35% of the time by giving them insufficient time to comply; because we don't know exactly how many children would have otherwise been successful, we might perhaps take from this a range of 51% to 86%. Remarkably, Shriver and Allen (1997) saw 98% of clinic-referred and nonreferred children aged 2 to 10 successfully follow through with directives given at least 14 seconds to do so (i.e., refraining from repeating the directive or engaging in physical guidance) with greater latency the younger the child; the difference in the referred versus nonreferred groups was in *whether*, not *when*, compliance occurred. The average compliance latency was 6 seconds.

Strain and colleagues (1983) looked at kindergarten through third-grade classrooms and reported compliance rates from 72% (the average compliance rate for teacher-rated maladjusted students) to 90% (the average for well-adjusted students). Whiting and Edwards (1988) reported a 72% to 82% compliance rate across nationalities with lower rates found for younger children and for boys. Brumfeld and Roberts (1998) reported an average compliance rate of 78% for a group of 4- and 5-year-olds but only 32% for a group of 2- and 3-year-olds. *Noncompliance* rates of 17% (Jacobs et al., 2000) and 8% to 54% (Rodriguez, Thompson, & Baynham, 2010) have been reported; the inverse of these figures would suggest expected compliance rates between 46% and 92%.

A synthesis of these data yields expected compliance rates ranging from 32% and 98% with known mediating variables being age and sex of the child and the amount of time the child is given to follow through. At the extremes of the compliance rate continuum are 100% which at least for toddlers may reflect physical abuse (Crittenden & DiLalla, 1988) and 0% to 60% which is low enough (Forehand, 1977) to predict impairment (McMahon & Forehand, 2003) as well as conduct problems in adolescence (Shriver & Allen, 2008). I regard a 70% compliance rate within 10 seconds of the directive as the norm for children ages 4 and up and a worthwhile and attainable treatment goal.

Treatment of Behavioral Noncompliance

Behavioral compliance is an operant shaped through interaction with the world (Nevin, 1996). Noncompliance, then, may also be seen as a product of the child's learning history – one in which contingencies of reinforcement have not sufficiently supported following directives. When compliance is low, caregivers are shaped into repeating themselves, providing rationales for why it is important to follow directives, and offering advance notice. Repeating directives over and over again may come to function as a punisher which tends to train the child to avoid the punishment and the punisher and engage in countercontrol (Sidman, 2001; Skinner, 1953). The child might also tune the parent out. Logic would lead us to believe providing rationales and advance notice would help, but these have been shown to be ineffective (Wilder *et al.*, 2010; Wilder, Nicholson, & Allison, 2010).

Setting events generally have been shown to affect compliance rate (Call *et al.*, 2004) given that they may represent motivating operations (Piazza *et al.*, 1997). Manipulating many of these variables produces treatment packages which may be preventative or therapeutic and individualized by behavioral function (one might suspect noncompliance to always be maintained by negative reinforcement in the form of escape and avoidance, but some studies have demonstrated an attention function, e.g., Reimers *et al.*, 1993, and Rodriguez, Thompson, & Baynham, 2010; see also Hurd *et al.*, 2023).

The behavioral parent training (BPT) literature is heavy on compliance building, and recommended procedures (see Barkley, 2013; Chorpita & Weisz, 2009; McMahon & Forehand, 2003; and McNeil & Hembree-Kigin, 2010) work quite well for children up to age 8 or so (Schroeder & Smith-Boydston, 2017). Additional treatment components are often necessary for older children, such as token reinforcement and contingency contracting, and offering the family guidance as to how to improve communication and problem-solving skills such as respectful negotiation (Barkley, 2013; Barkley & Robin, 2014; Shriver & Allen, 2008).

Interventions known to improve behavioral compliance and reviewed below include time-in, effective directive delivery, errorless compliance training, three-step guided compliance, reward programs, time-out, and the daily behavior report card. Many of these are typically combined into a treatment package for families. It is sometimes important to preface for caregivers who are relatively indulgent at intake that the point of working on behavioral compliance is not to produce robots or docile children, but to increase coachability and improve family life (McMahon & Forehand, 2003; Risley, Clark, & Cataldo, 1976) as well as offer a training simulation of the conditions found outside of the home, such as the classroom and sports field, and eventually, the workplace. I routinely advise that children not be told to be "leaders" (caregivers commonly say this to caution against peer pressure, but this could be communicated more directly) but instead to be excellent followers of the legitimate authority figures in their lives until adulthood. The high school football coach whose players make leadership easy is able to efficiently shape their skills, making it more likely the team will win some games. The classroom teacher whose students make leadership easy is able to efficiently teach the day's lessons. Likewise, the caregiver whose child makes leadership easy is able to teach the child anything, which in turn leads to healthy family dynamics and better outcomes for the child through the years.

In any event, when clinicians find themselves addressing behavioral noncompliance it is likely to co-occur with either a mutually coercive family dynamic and lots of yelling in the home, or in the case of noncompliance only at school, a home environment that places few demands on the child. Caregivers benefit from being told on the front end that we must move from coercion and control to guidance and support, from emotionally reactive correction to loving, proactive coaching and mentoring, and sometimes, from offering the child a role in family life other than that of consumer. The interventions reviewed below help to move in these directions.

I routinely prescribe time-in and differential attending, effective directive delivery, errorless compliance training, and guided compliance procedures, finding such a package sufficient for effectively improving behavioral compliance rates to at least 70% (primarily measured by caregiver report) in most cases. My reliance on reward programs and exclusionary time-out procedures, if used at all, tends to be short-lived per case. Caregivers are urged to refrain from repeating themselves or issuing verbal heads-up or contingent consequence warnings, reminders, or rationales within the moment of directive delivery. The child should awaken each day without access to privileges (e.g., screen electronics) and earn them contingent upon sufficient cooperation and respect. Generalization of treatment gains to the classroom is seen in nearly all cases also involving noncompliance with teacher directives, and in those cases in which treatment effects fail to naturally generalize, the daily behavior report card tends to do the trick. These treatment components are discussed in more detail below.

Time-In

Time-in, conceptualized as the opposing condition to that intended by the time-out intervention instead involving noncontingent social reinforcement in the relative absence of inappropriate behavior (Christophersen, 1988; Ford *et al.*, 2001; Roberts *et al.*, 2008), has been demonstrated to improve compliance. A structured version of time-in is represented by the Child's Game (Forehand & Scarboro, 1975; Johnson & Lobitz, 1974; McMahon & Forehand, 2003), a daily 10- to 15-minute free-play session held at home by caregivers with their children during which the child plays with a favored toy or activity (ideally Lego, cars, coloring, or similar activity which allows creativity and goal-directed play; this would not include screen electronics use). During this interval, the caregiver offers the child his or her full attention, offers a fun play-by-play narrative of what the child is doing, praises anything praiseworthy, and completely refrains from issuing directives, corrections, lessons, or questions. No demands are placed on the child during this time, and every second is meant to be mutually rewarding. The caregiver follows rather than leads the child and ignores any problem behavior. The *Child's Game* is so named as the counterpoint to the *Parent's Game*, the remainder of the day during which the caregiver leads the child (McMahon & Forehand, 2003).

Effective Directive Delivery

Effective directive delivery is another important component of BPT packages. This entails augmenting the stimulus control of directives by reducing distraction and increasing proximity; saying the child's name and looking into his or her eyes; issuing single-step and not multistep directives; offering sufficient time for follow-through; being polite and respectful yet still using a firm voice; issuing direct, authoritative statements rather than requests; using "do" rather than "don't" directives; using clear, age-appropriate vocabulary; and remaining silent instead of repeating the directive once issued (Everett *et al.*, 2005; McMahon & Forehand, 2003; McNeil & Hembree-Kigin, 2010; Morris, Conway, & Goetz, 2021; Ndoro *et al.*, 2006; Tarbox *et al.*, 2007).

Errorless Compliance Training

Directives may be categorized as high-probability (or "high-p", meaning directives that are likely to be followed) and low-probability (or "low-p", meaning directives that are unlikely to be followed) for a given child. High-p directives may then be issued to the exclusion of lower-p directives for a time, to make success with following directives more likely to in turn allow the child to more easily and frequently contact contingent reinforcement with following directives. High-p and low-p directives are then crossfaded. Such an approach, which also incorporates differential attending (i.e., offering contingent acknowledgment of appropriate behavior while placing problem behavior on extinction) and effective directive delivery, has been termed *errorless compliance training* (Ducharme, 1996) and has been shown to generalize to untreated settings like the classroom (Cavell *et al.*, 2018). A variation of this approach involves issuing a series of high-p directives followed by lower-p directives all in one sitting which is reported to produce what may be called *behavioral momentum* (Mace *et al.*, 1988; Nevin, 1996). Contingent reinforcement is a necessary component, however, with more momentum resulting from more reinforcement (Mace *et al.*, 1988). Timeout has sometimes been a necessary supplemental component (Rortvedt & Miltenberger, 1994).

Three-Step Guided Compliance

The three-step guided compliance method described in Chapter 4 represents another procedural consideration for improving behavioral compliance. To reiterate, it involves issuing a verbal directive (Step 1) and in the absence of compliance escalating to the issuance of prompts from least to most intrusive (i.e., modeling, Step 2, followed by physical prompting, Step 3). Behavioral skills training, also described in Chapter 4, involves offering instructions, modeling successful responding, having the learner rehearse that successful responding in the presence of discriminative stimuli, and offering feedback.

Reward Programs

The effective use of rewards in professional practice is more involved than commonly believed. Children whose problem behavior quickly resolves with the use of a simple reward contingency implemented by caregivers or teachers may be said to have had a motivational deficit. We in practice tend to not meet these children because they generally don't need us. That little added incentive does the trick.

Sometimes out there, however, reward programs fail, likely due to the selected reward not serving as a reinforcer, or perhaps more likely, the problem is not a deficit of motivation but one of skill. If the child doesn't know how to do it, no amount of reward will matter. These are the kids that find us. Regarding these cases, I routinely explain that rewards, in clinical practice, should be relied upon only after 1) relevant skills have been taught based on consideration of behavioral function, 2) behavioral expectations have been clearly communicated, 3) the reward criteria may be met without excessive required effort or frustration, and 4) an apparent motivational deficit nonetheless remains.

Expectations may be clearly communicated in any or a combination of the following examples, also serving as prompts, and while heeding effective directive delivery considerations:

- Brief, encouraging daily "morning meetings" between caregiver or teacher and the child, enthusiastically reminding the child what is expected today
- Verbal reminders for a short while, to be faded out
- Visual reminders (e.g., posted picture schedules, rules, bulleted task-analyzed steps)
- For older children, texts and pre-programmed alerts on their screen electronic devices
- Contingency contracting

Contingent rewards can take virtually any form, from recognition to a privilege, trinket, or treat. I generally advise against trinkets or treats, however, stating my preference for rewards that don't cost us much or require a last-minute trip to the store. A reward menu, designed like a restaurant menu, may be used, laying out all possible rewards to be chosen from each day which increases the likelihood of the reward serving as a reinforcer; when a reward is earned, it's the menu that is earned, allowing the child to choose what looks best at the moment. A token system is an option, involving the earning of tokens (e.g., points, stickers, poker chips) to be traded later for a desired reward or access to the reward menu. A dot-to-dot reward system described by Christophersen and Friman (2010) is particularly easy to design and implement and for the child to understand: dots are drawn around a picture of an object or activity the child desires, and successful practice of a skill earns a dot to be connected. When all dots are connected, the child immediately earns the item depicted. In any event, care must be taken to ensure the selected reward functions as a reinforcer (see the Reinforcer Identification section of Chapter 3) and continues to serve as one over time. And, the simpler the reward system, the more likely it is to be maintained over time.

Perhaps a more naturalistic and sustainable approach to reward use, however, is to make preferred activities contingent upon meeting preset criteria each day (e.g., requiring chores to be done without verbal prompting, siblings to get along, general cooperation with caregivers, no negative comments from the teacher, and homework completed, prior to access to videogaming; moreover, failure to reliably and gracefully relinquish the gaming device when expected precludes gaming the following day). This is essentially designing the day's flow based on the Premack principle, and perhaps represents a proper default authoritative management system. Also, nearly universal reinforcers for children are caregiver availability and responsiveness, and enjoying some measure of control over their world and being able to make some decisions; caregivers would do well to, as a rule, make these contingent upon meeting expectations moment by moment.

Yet another important consideration is that behavioral function of a problem behavior likely serves as a more potent reinforcer at the moment than any reward chosen – the greatest implication being that offering a functionally equivalent prosocial behavior to replace the problem behavior may be a more effective strategy than designing a reward program to solve the problem. As discussed in Chapter 3, function-based intervention is superior to old-school behavior modification and reflects the evolution of our science and practice. Reward programs, again, should only be considered once behavioral function has.

An oft-heard argument against reward use is that it is tantamount to bribery. "I don't want to bribe my kid" is usually the line. Indeed, *do that and you get this* is how bribes work. But here's the question: in using rewards, are we attempting to have our clients engage in an illegal or unethical activity, or engage in a skill that will bring about more success for everyone involved? If the former, then yes, it's a bribe. If the latter, then it's an incentive, and likely a short-term one at that (those not finding this distinction compelling may wish to voluntarily forgo their paychecks, given that they are being bribed to show up for work every day).

The clinician may also be asked whether rewards indeed harm natural motivation for what is being rewarded. It is important for the clinician to understand where this notion comes from and how to address it. That rewards may be harmful appears to stem from a line of mentalistic research beginning in the 1970s (e.g., Deci, 1971; Lepper, Greene, & Nisbett, 1973). Behavior analysts have since weighed in with commentary and data, and demonstrated there to be little concern particularly as employed by behavior analysts in practice (see, for example, Eisenberger & Cameron, 1996; McGinnis, Friman, & Carlyon, 1999; and Reitman, 1998a, 1998b).

Time-Out

Time-out, or more accurately, "time-out from positive reinforcement," has appeared for decades in the behavior-analytic literature (e.g., Baer, 1962; Donaldson & Vollmer, 2011; Rortvedt & Miltenberger, 1994) and, in the historical context of being an alternative to corporal punishment, is recommended by pediatricians (Scholer, Nix, & Patterson, 2006). Most caregivers use it, but ineffectively so (Riley et al., 2017). Time-out may be used as a consequence for problem behavior geared for attention or some tangible item, and may also be used when the child is so emotional and unreasonable as to need some time alone to calm down (Chacko et al., 2018). All effective time-out procedures are variations on the common theme of removing access to reinforcement contingent upon the occurrence of a target problem behavior. Critically, time-out procedures may have the intended effect on behavior only in cases in which the child will be removed from a time-in condition (Mathews et al., 1987; Shriver & Allen, 1996).

Variations from least to most intrusive include *non-exclusionary*, such as with planned ignoring or removal of a specific reinforcing stimulus such as pausing a video, *exclusionary*, such as physically moving the child away from the action, and *isolation*, such as physically moving the child to his bedroom (O'Handley, Olmi, & Kennedy, 2019). A commonly recommended time-out duration is one minute for every year of age (Anastopoulos & Farley, 2003). As to release from time-out, a longstanding recommendation has been that once that predetermined amount of time has elapsed, the child may be released as long as there is an absence of problem behavior to avoid accidentally reinforcing it, but Donaldson and Vollmer (2011) demonstrated such contingent release to be likely unnecessary.

As a general principle (and consistent with the Ethics Code for Behavior Analysts Standards 2.14 and 2.15; Behavior Analyst Certification Board, 2020), reinforcement procedures should be considered prior to time-out and other punishment procedures. Notably, time-out may be unnecessary given a combination of time-in and effective directive delivery (Ford et al., 2001). A combination of reinforcement and punishment procedures is, however, often required for behavior change, and in such cases, the least intrusive effective procedures should be considered.

Daily Behavior Report Card

The daily behavior report card, also known as the school-home note, is a means of communication between the classroom and the home allowing the caregiver to provide positive or negative consequences after school for school-based behavior. The teacher and caregiver agree on one or more target behaviors occurring in the classroom and the teacher then provides feedback to the caregiver immediately after school, ideally before the child arrives home. Teacher and caregiver adherence with this intervention is likely to be higher the simpler the card, so using a binary rating of "met" or "did not meet" expectations per target behavior may be preferred. Wherever the overall standard is set, the child either enjoys privileges after school or no privileges with an early bedtime, for example. Token reinforcement is an option here as well. This simple intervention enjoys strong empirical support as a treatment for problem behavior in the classroom (Iznardo *et al.*, 2020).

Key Takeaways from this Chapter

- Behavioral noncompliance, or failure to initiate within 10 seconds the follow-through of a directive issued by a caregiver or other legitimate authority figure, is a common problem of childhood which predicts mental health diagnosis and the development of many other problem behaviors that impede social, academic, and other important areas of functioning. Improving compliance improves coachability and decreases problem behavior. For these reasons, it is considered a clinical metafactor to be prioritized in treatment.
- Typical compliance rates appear to range from 32% and 98% depending on the age of the child and the amount of time the child is given to follow through. Generally, the younger the child and the less time the child is given to comply before the directive is repeated, the lower the compliance rate. Compliance rates under 60% predict current and future impairment. The author regards a 70% compliance rate within 10 seconds of the directive as the norm for children ages 4 and up and a worthwhile and attainable treatment goal.
- Behavioral treatment for noncompliance generally involves manipulation of antecedent and consequent variables to occasion and shape compliance. The behavioral parent training literature supports compliance building via implementation of time-in, effective directive

delivery, errorless compliance training, time-out, guided compliance procedures, and at times a contingency management system addressing school-based problem behavior. Reinforcement procedures should be used before punishment procedures (e.g., time-out), as the latter may ultimately prove unnecessary.

• A reward program, if used, should follow the acquisition of relevant skills to be rewarded, clearly communicated expectations, an indication that reward criteria are reasonable, function-based intervention, and continued demonstrated need for a reward component. Reward programs as designed and implemented by behavior analysts do not represent "bribery" and do not hurt natural motivation.

References

Achenbach, T. M., & Edelbrock, C. S. (1981). *Behavioral problems and competencies reported by parents of normal and disturbed children aged four through sixteen* (Monographs of the Society for Research in Child Development, No. 188). Society for Research in Child Development.

Anastopoulos, A. D., & Farley, S. E. (2003). A cognitive-behavioral training program for parents of children with attention-deficit/hyperactivity disorder. In A. E. Kazdin & J. R. Weisz (Eds.), *Evidence-based psychotherapies for children and adolescents* (pp. 187–203). Guilford.

Baer, D. M. (1962). Laboratory control of thumbsucking by withdrawal and re-presentation of reinforcement. *Journal of the Experimental Analysis of Behavior, 5*, 525–528.

Barkley, R. A. (2013). *Defiant children: A clinician's manual for assessment and parent training* (3rd ed.). Guilford.

Barkley, R. A., & Robin, A. L. (2014). *Defiant teens: A clinician's manual for assessment and family intervention* (2nd ed.). Guilford.

Behavior Analyst Certification Board (2020). *Ethics code for behavior analysts.* https://bcba.com/wp-content/ethics-code-for-behavior-analysts/

Brumfeld, B. D., & Roberts, M. W. (1998). A comparison of two measurements of child compliance with normal preschool children. *Journal of Clinical Child Psychology, 27*, 109–116.

Call, N. A., Wacker, D. P., Ringdahl, J. E., Cooper-Brown, L. J., & Boelter, E. W. (2004). An assessment of antecedent events influencing noncompliance in an outpatient clinic. *Journal of Applied Behavior Analysis, 37*, 145–158.

Cavell, H. J., Radley, K. C., Dufrene, B. A., Tingstrom, D. H., Ness, E. A., & Murphy, A. N. (2018). The effects of errorless compliance training on children in home and school settings. *Behavioral Interventions, 33*, 391–402.

Chacko, A., Allan, C. C., Uderman, J., Cornwell, M., Anderson, L., & Chimiklis, A. (2018). Training parents of youth with ADHD. In R. A. Barkley (Ed.), *Attention-deficit hyperactivity disorder: A handbook for diagnosis and treatment* (4th ed., pp. 513–536). Guilford.

Charlop, M. H., Parrish, J. M., Fenton, L. R., & Cataldo, M. F. (1987). Evaluation of hospital-based outpatient pediatric psychology services. *Journal of Pediatric Psychology, 12,* 485–503.

Chorpita, B. F., & Weisz, J. R. (2009). *Modular approach to therapy for children with anxiety, depression, trauma, or conduct problems (MATCH-ADTC).* PracticeWise.

Christophersen, E. R. (1988). *Little people: Guidelines for common sense child rearing* (3rd ed.). Overland.

Christophersen, E. R., & Friman, P. C. (2010). *Elimination disorders in children and adolescents.* Hogrefe.

Crittenden, P. M., & DiLalla, D. L. (1988). Compulsive compliance: The development of an inhibitory coping strategy in infancy. *Journal of Abnormal Child Psychology, 16,* 585–599.

Deci, E. L. (1971). Effects of externally mediated rewards on intrinsic motivation. *Journal of Personality and Social Psychology, 18,* 105–115.

Donaldson, J. M., & Vollmer, T. R. (2011). An evaluation and comparison of time-out procedures with and without release contingencies. *Journal of Applied Behavior Analysis, 44,* 693–705.

Ducharme, J. M. (1996). Errorless compliance training: Optimizing clinical efficacy. *Behavior Modification, 20,* 259–280.

Eisenberger, R., & Cameron, J. (1996). Detrimental effects of reward: Reality or myth? *American Psychologist, 51,* 1153–1166.

Everett, G. E., Olmi, D. J., Edwards, R. P., & Tingstrom, D. H. (2005). The contributions of eye contact and contingent praise to effective instruction delivery in compliance training. *Education and Treatment of Children, 28,* 48–62.

Ford, A. D., Olmi, D. J., Edwards, R. P., & Tingstrom, D. H. (2001). The sequential introduction of compliance training components with elementary-aged children in general education classroom settings. *School Psychology Quarterly, 16,* 142–157.

Forehand, R. (1977). Child noncompliance to parental requests: Behavioral analysis and treatment. In M. Hersen, R. M. Eisler, & P. M. Miller (Eds.), *Progress in behavior modification* (Vol. 5, pp. 111–147). Academic.

Forehand, R., Gardner, H., & Roberts, M. (1978). Maternal response to child compliance and noncompliance: Some normative data. *Journal of Clinical Child Psychology, 7,* 121–124.

Forehand, R., & Scarboro, M. E. (1975). An analysis of children's oppositional behavior. *Journal of Abnormal Child Psychology, 3,* 27–31.

Friman, P. C. (2008). Primary care behavioral pediatrics. In M. Hersen & A. M. Gross (Eds.), *Handbook of clinical psychology* (Vol. 2; pp. 728–758). Wiley.

Hanley, G. P., Heal, N. A., Tiger, J. H., & Ingvarsson, E. T. (2007). Evaluation of a classwide teaching program for developing preschool life skills. *Journal of Applied Behavior Analysis, 40,* 277–300.

Hurd, A. M., Nercesian, S. J., Brown, K. R., & Visser, E. J. (2023). A systematic review on functional analysis of noncompliance. *Education and Treatment of Children, 46,* 45–58.

Iznardo, M., Rogers, M. A., Volpe, R. J., Labelle, P. R., & Robaey, P. (2020). The effectiveness of daily behavior report cards for children with ADHD: A meta-analysis. *Journal of Attention Disorders, 24,* 1623–1636.

Jacobs, J. R., Boggs, S. R., Eyberg, S. M., Edwards, D, Durning, P., Querido, J. G., McNeil, C. B., & Funderburk, B. W. (2000). Psychometric properties and reference point data for the Revised Edition of the School Observation Coding System. *Behavior Therapy, 31,* 695–712.

Johnson, S. M., & Lobitz, G. K. (1974). Parental manipulation of child behavior in home observations. *Journal of Applied Behavior Analysis, 7,* 23–31.

Kalb, L. M., & Loeber, R. (2003). Child disobedience and noncompliance: A review. *Pediatrics, 111,* 641–652.

Keenan, K., Shaw, D., Delliquadri, E., Giovanelli, J., & Walsh, B. (1998). Evidence for the continuity of early problem behaviors: Application of a developmental model. *Journal of Abnormal Child Psychology, 26,* 441–454.

Lepper, M. R., Greene, D., & Nisbett, R. E. (1973). Undermining children's intrinsic interest with extrinsic reward: A test of the "overjustification" hypothesis. *Journal of Personality and Social Psychology, 28,* 129–137.

Mace, F. C., Hock, M. L., Lalli, J. S., West, B. J., Belfiore, P., Pinter, E., & Brown, D. K. (1988). Behavioral momentum in the treatment of noncompliance. *Journal of Applied Behavior Analysis, 21,* 123–141.

Martens, B. K., & Kelly, S. Q. (1993). A behavioral analysis of effective teaching. *School Psychology Quarterly, 8,* 10–26.

Mathews, J. R., Friman, P. C., Barone, V. J., Ross, L. V., & Christophersen, E. R. (1987). Decreasing dangerous infant behavior through parent instruction. *Journal of Applied Behavior Analysis, 20,* 165–169.

McGinnis, J. C., Friman, P. C., & Carlyon, W. D. (1999). The effect of token rewards on "intrinsic" motivation for doing math. *Journal of Applied Behavior Analysis, 32,* 375–379.

McMahon, R. J., & Forehand, R. L. (2003). *Helping the noncompliant child: Family-based treatment for oppositional behavior* (2nd ed.). Guilford.

McNeil, C. B., & Hembree-Kigin, T. L. (2010). *Parent-child interaction therapy* (2nd ed.). Springer.

Morris, C., Conway, A. A., & Goetz, D. B. (2021). A review of effective strategies for parent-delivered instruction. *Behavior Analysis in Practice, 14,* 513–522.

Ndoro, V. W., Hanley, G. P., Tiger, J. H., & Heal, N. A. (2006). A descriptive assessment of instruction-based interactions in the preschool classroom. *Journal of Applied Behavior Analysis, 39,* 79–90.

Nergaard, S. K., & Couto, K. C. (2021). Effects of reinforcement and response-cost history on instructional control. *Journal of the Experimental Analysis of Behavior, 115,* 679–701.

Nevin, J. A. (1996). The momentum of compliance. *Journal of Applied Behavior Analysis, 29,* 535–547.

O'Handley, R. D., Olmi, D. J., & Kennedy, A. (2019). Time-out procedures in school settings. In K. C. Radley & E. H. Dart (Eds.), *Handbook of behavioral interventions in schools: Multi-tiered systems of support* (pp. 482–500). Oxford.

Parrish, J. M., Cataldo, M. F., Kolko, D. J., Neef, N. A., & Egel, A. L. (1986). Experimental analysis of response covariation among compliant and inappropriate behaviors. *Journal of Applied Behavior Analysis, 19,* 241–254.

Piazza, C. C., Contrucci, S. A., Hanley, G. P., & Fisher, W. W. (1997). Nondirective prompting and noncontingent reinforcement in the treatment of destructive behavior during hygiene routines. *Journal of Applied Behavior Analysis, 30,* 705–708.

Reimers, T. M., Wacker, D. P., Cooper, L. J., Sasso, G. M., Berg, W. K., & Steege, M. W. (1993). Assessing the functional properties of noncompliant behavior in an outpatient setting. *Child & Family Behavior Therapy, 19,* 1–15.

Reitman, D. (1998a). The real and imagined harmful effects of rewards: Implications for clinical practice. *Journal of Behavior Therapy and Experimental Psychiatry, 29,* 101–113.

Reitman, D. (1998b). Punished by misunderstanding: A critical evaluation of Kohn's *Punished by Rewards* and its implications for behavioral interventions with children. *The Behavior Analyst, 21,* 143–157.

Riley, A. R., Wagner, D. V., Tudor, M. E., Zuckerman, K. E., & Freeman, K. A. (2017). A survey of parents' perceptions and use of time-out compared to empirical evidence. *Academic Pediatrics, 17,* 168–175.

Risley, T. R., Clark, H. B., & Cataldo, M. F. (1976). Behavioral technology for the normal middle-class family. In E. J. Mash, L. A. Hamerlynck, & L. C. Handy (Eds.), *Behavior modification and families* (pp. 34–60). Brunner/Mazel.

Roberts, D. S., Tingstrom, D. H., Olmi, D. J., & Bellipanni, K. D. (2008). Positive antecedent and consequent components in child compliance training. *Behavior Modification, 32,* 21–38.

Rodriguez, N. W., Thompson, R. H., & Baynham, T. Y. (2010). Assessment of the relative effects of attention and escape on noncompliance. *Journal of Applied Behavior Analysis, 43,* 143–147.

Rortvedt, A. K., & Miltenberger, R. G. (1994). Analysis of a high-probability instructional sequence and timeout in the treatment of child noncompliance. *Journal of Applied Behavior Analysis, 27,* 327–330.

Scholer, S. J., Nix, R. L., & Patterson, B. (2006). Gaps in pediatricians' advice to parents regarding early childhood aggression. *Clinical Pediatrics, 45,* 23–28.

Schroeder, C. S., & Smith-Boydston, J. M. (2017). *Assessment and treatment of childhood problems: A clinician's guide* (3rd ed.). Guilford.

Shriver, M. D., & Allen, K. D. (1996). The time-out grid: A guide to effective discipline. *School Psychology Quarterly, 11,* 67–74.

Shriver, M. D., & Allen, K. D. (1997). Defining child noncompliance: An examination of temporal parameters. *Journal of Applied Behavior Analysis, 30,* 173–176.

Shriver, M. D., & Allen, K. D. (2008). *Working with parents of noncompliant children: A guide to evidence-based parent training for practitioners and students.* American Psychological Association.

Sidman, M. (2001). *Coercion and its fallout (rev. ed.).* Authors Cooperative.

Skinner, B. F. (1953). *Science and human behavior.* Free Press.

Strain, P. S., Lambert, D. L., Kerr, M. M., Stagg, V., & Lenkner, D. A. (1983). Naturalistic assessment of children's compliance to teachers' requests and consequences for compliance. *Journal of Applied Behavior Analysis, 16,* 243–249.

Tarbox, R. S. F., Wallace, M. D., Penrod, B., & Tarbox, J. (2007). Effects of three-step prompting on compliance with caregiver requests. *Journal of Applied Behavior Analysis, 40,* 703–706.

Watson, T. S., Foster, N., & Friman, P. C. (2006). Treatment adherence in children and adolescents. In W. T. O'Donohue & E. R. Levensky (Eds.), *Promoting treatment adherence: A practical handbook for health care providers* (pp. 343–351). Sage.

Whiting, B. B., & Edwards, C. P. (1988). *Children of different worlds: The formation of social behavior.* Harvard.

Wilder, D. A., Allison, J., Nicholson, K., Abellon, O. E., & Saulnier, R. (2010). Further evaluation of antecedent interventions on compliance: The effects of rationales to increase compliance among preschoolers. *Journal of Applied Behavior Analysis, 43,* 601–613.

Wilder, D. A., Nicholson, K., & Allison, J. (2010). An evaluation of advance notice to increase compliance among preschoolers. *Journal of Applied Behavior Analysis, 43,* 751–755.

Poor Toleration of Denial and Delay

8

A complementary life skill to behavioral compliance is the graceful acceptance of the decisions of authority figures. Compliance is about increasing desired behavior, whereas acceptance is about prevention or abatement of undesired behavior, and the termination of a preferred activity, all via verbal direction. Both are required for instructional control and a child benefiting from the wise words and direction of those who love him or her most. Acceptance of decisions, or relative lack thereof, is therefore considered another clinical metafactor.

Nonacceptance of decisions may be conceptualized as delay intolerance. When a child mands, the caregiver may respond with something along the lines of "no" or "not yet." The fact that the child mands at all is evidence of its being historically reinforced. Denying a child's request places that mand on extinction, which in turn may produce an extinction burst. Extinction bursting from delay intolerance is the problem for caregivers in such a scenario.

In the behavioral literature, delay tolerance is discussed primarily in the context of reinforcement schedule thinning in programming for maintenance during functional communication training (FCT). Of all possible thinning schedules including delay schedules, chain schedules, multiple schedules, and response restriction (see Hagopian, Boelter, & Jarmolowicz, 2011), the most common in nature are delay schedules, or gradual increases in the delay between mand and reinforcement delivery, and they also appear most likely to produce extinction bursting following delays of under a minute (Ghaemmaghami, Hanley, & Jessel, 2016).

DOI: 10.4324/9781003371281-9

Another way of conceptualizing nonacceptance of decisions is by viewing it in the colloquial terms of impulsivity or poor self-control. Neef, Bicard, and Endo (2001) defined *impulsivity* as "choices between concurrently available response alternatives that produce smaller immediate reinforcers rather than larger delayed reinforcers" and its opposite, *self-control*, as "choices that produce relatively greater yields at a later point in time" (p. 397). Similarly, Binder, Dixon, and Ghezzi (2000) noted, "There are many situations in which a person is asked to select between a small immediate reinforcer and a larger delayed reinforcer of unknown delay duration. Choices for the small immediate option in these situations are termed *impulsive*, and choices for the larger delayed option are termed *self-control*" (p. 233, italics in original). A classic study on delay of gratification was the Stanford marshmallow experiment (Mischel, Ebbesen, & Zeiss, 1972); children of preschool age were each given an opportunity to immediately eat a marshmallow or to wait 15 minutes to eat two marshmallows. Follow-ups decades later (Mischel, Shoda, & Peake, 1988; Shoda, Mischel, & Peake, 1990) found the children's choices predictive of future outcomes such as competence ratings and SAT scores. Perhaps nonacceptance of decisions is analogous to opting for the first marshmallow. Self-control may be increased (and impulsivity decreased) via gradually increasing the delay to the larger reward (Neef, Bicard, & Endo, 2001). For example, Schweitzer and Sulzer-Azaroff (1988), with children nominated for impulsivity, increased the probability of their choosing larger, more delayed rewards over smaller, more immediate reinforcers this way.

All things considered, the following guidelines are offered in efforts to improve a child's toleration of denial and delay:

- Explicitly teach what is expected. Tierney and Green (2022), for example, task analyzed nearly 200 life skills, with Accepting Decisions of Authority being one of them. Their recommended steps for this particular skill are 1) look at the person, 2) listen carefully to the person's decision without interrupting, 3) avoid arguing or becoming angry, 4) when you have the opportunity to speak, use a calm voice, 5) acknowledge the decision by saying, "Okay" or "I understand," and 6) if appropriate, request a reason or disagree appropriately at a later time. Teaching this, however, could be as simple as explaining, "When I say no, I need you to say 'okay'."
- Contingency-based delays appear to be more effective than time-based delays for increasing delay tolerance (Ghaemmaghami, Hanley, & Jessel, 2016; Hanley et al., 2014). That is, delivery of reinforcement is

made contingent upon the child making a toleration response (e.g., saying "okay") as well as engagement in leisure items meantime.

- Relatedly, and taking a page from Hanley and his team, I devised a teaching procedure involving caregivers guarding access to preferred items for a few weeks, instructing and requiring respectful manding for those items, hearing "no" and immediately responding with a toleration response (saying "okay"), and caregivers immediately changing their minds and enthusiastically granting the request. The idea here is to establish stimulus control for the toleration response. Once acceptance becomes a habit pattern (e.g., after a few weeks of successful trials), preferred items are no longer proactively withheld and caregivers quickly fade their change of mind rate from around 90% to 20% which then remains in place. Nonacceptance throughout is placed on extinction. Note that accepting *no* for an answer may be made easier by first training *not yet* as an answer. The no condition may be seen as a much longer delay of reinforcement than the not-yet condition. The not-yet condition should be trained with very brief delays (e.g., five seconds) at first.
- A recent study on delay of gratification found that preschool children make decisions at least partly based on the probability of reputational improvement or damage resulting from their choices (Ma *et al.*, 2020). Caregivers may consider incorporating statements during training reflecting the positive impressions that graceful acceptance and patient waiting make on others.
- As a good parenting rule, children should generally earn what they want, if only by asking nicely and demonstrating the ability to wait a bit.

Key Takeaways from this Chapter

- Poor toleration of denial and delay, or nonacceptance of decisions, is a problem for many families and along with behavioral compliance is required for adequate instructional control. It is therefore considered another clinical metafactor.
- Delay schedules are the most common thinning schedule found in nature yet represent the one most likely to produce rapid extinction bursting. A delay schedule is represented by gradual increases in the delay between mand and reinforcement delivery. Delay tolerance may be more easily improved with the use of contingency-based delays, represented by the delivery of reinforcement contingent upon the child

making a toleration response (e.g., saying "okay") as well as engagement in leisure items meantime.

• The colloquial terms *impulsivity* and *poor self-control* may be viewed as another set of names for behavior resulting in smaller immediate reinforcement instead of larger delayed reward given the choice. This phenomenon has been studied under the construct of delay of gratification, such as in the Stanford marshmallow experiment. Such choice behavior may be shaped via gradually increasing the delay to the larger reward. Explicitly teaching and shaping a tolerance response as a replacement behavior, placing protest behavior on extinction, and offering plenty of positive practice improves toleration of denial and delay.

References

Binder, L. M., Dixon, M. R., & Ghezzi, P. M. (2000). A procedure to teach self-control to children with attention deficit hyperactivity disorder. *Journal of Applied Behavior Analysis, 33*, 233–237.

Ghaemmaghami, M., Hanley, G. P., & Jessel, J. (2016). Contingencies promote delay tolerance. *Journal of Applied Behavior Analysis, 49*, 548–575.

Hagopian, L. P., Boelter, E. W., Jarmolowicz, D. P. (2011). Reinforcement schedule thinning following functional communication: Review and recommendations. *Behavior Analysis in Practice, 4*, 4–16.

Hanley, G. P., Jin, C. S., Vanselow, N. R., & Hanratty, L. A. (2014). Producing meaningful improvements in problem behavior of children with autism via synthesized analyses and treatments. *Journal of Applied Behavior Analysis, 47*, 16–36.

Ma, F., Zeng, D., Xu, F., Compton, B. J., & Heyman, G. D. (2020). Delay of gratification as reputation management. *Psychological Science, 31*, 1174–1182.

Mischel, W., Ebbesen, E. B., & Zeiss, A. R. (1972). Cognitive and attentional mechanisms in delay of gratification. *Journal of Personality and Social Psychology, 21*, 204–218.

Mischel, W., Shoda, Y., & Peake, P. K. (1988). The nature of adolescent competencies predicted by preschool delay of gratification. *Journal of Personality and Social Psychology, 54*, 687–696.

Neef, N. A., Bicard, D. F., & Endo, S. (2001). Assessment of impulsivity and the development of self-control in students with attention deficit hyperactivity disorder. *Journal of Applied Behavior Analysis, 34*, 397–408.

Schweitzer, J. B., & Sulzer-Azaroff, B. (1988). Self-control: Teaching tolerance for delay in impulsive children. *Journal of the Experimental Analysis of Behavior, 50*, 173–186.

Shoda, Y., Mischel, W., & Peake, P. K. (1990). Predicting adolescent cognitive and self-regulatory competencies from preschool delay of gratification: Identifying diagnostic conditions. *Developmental Psychology, 26*, 978–986.

Tierney, J., & Green, E. (2022). *Teaching social skills to youth: An easy-to-follow guide to teaching 196 basic to complex life skills* (4th ed). Boys Town.

Poor Self-Advocacy Skills 9

If the metafactor of toleration for denial and delay is about the child accepting no, the metafactor of self-advocacy is about the child *saying* no, when appropriate. It is about the child otherwise speaking up to ask for a break, for help, or for a desired item. Strong self-advocacy skills include the ability and unprompted initiation of requesting clarification, sticking up for self and others, offering constructive feedback, and reporting peers' problem behavior to adults in addition to appropriately disagreeing, requesting attention, requesting items from peers, asking for alone time to cool down from being upset, and asking for help or advice.

Effective self-advocacy may be viewed as a repertoire of appropriate verbal mands, and the younger the child and the more severe the presentation, the less likely the child possesses this repertoire. Manding as a skill set may be considered a cusp (Costa & Pelaez, 2014; Hixson, 2004) which tends to open the world to the child, while also serving as a repertoire of conflict prevention skills (e.g., requesting a toy held by another child instead of simply lunging and grabbing for it not only gets the toy but potentially earns a playmate instead of causing a scene). Indeed, teaching mands is known to significantly reduce problem behavior (Drifke, Tiger, & Lillie, 2020; Hanley *et al.*, 2007; Tiger, Hanley, & Bruzek, 2008).

Some examples of inadequate self-advocacy skills and their remediation are offered below.

- A preschooler constantly verbally interrupts her caregiver when on the phone or in conversation with another adult. The caregiver is offered

DOI: 10.4324/9781003371281-10

guidance in teaching the child to stand a few feet away and raise her index finger as a proper gestural mand for attention. The caregiver now responds immediately to the gesture either by responding verbally or gesturally signaling that she must take her turn and wait for another few seconds.

- Two preschool-age siblings constantly verbally and physically fight over desired items. The caregiver is offered guidance in teaching proper manding for the item (e.g., keeping hands and voice down, and politely asking for the item) and choreographing the sibling's appropriate response to the new manding (e.g., "Ok, here, but I want it back soon").
- A school-age child is told to take out the trash but believes this directive to be unfair given that his sibling never has to do it. He frequently complains in a whiny and sometimes defiant manner which escalates the situation. There is already much yelling in the home and this occasions more. The caregiver is offered guidance in teaching the skill of appropriate disagreeing, which entails a) immediately saying okay and following through, b) waiting a few minutes, and c) respectfully asking the caregiver if they can talk about that chore for next time. The caregiver should reinforce this new approach by agreeing to sit and talk and encourage the child to propose an alternative. Perhaps the siblings could take turns taking the trash out from now on.
- An introverted school-age child is struggling in math and is not completing his math homework. His grades are falling and his caregivers have confiscated his phone as a punishment. However, this is not a motivational problem but a skill problem; he doesn't know what he's doing in math. His teacher hasn't offered additional help but he hasn't asked for it either. The caregiver is offered guidance in training him to ask for help both at school and at home, with sanctions lifted for proper manding for help and improved grades.
- A preteen is habitually responding irritably to family members. The caregiver is offered guidance in teaching the child to a) label the predominant emotion he is feeling, and b) ask for some alone time, for someone to just listen for a moment, or for some guidance.

The clinician may include the child directly during the initial assessment as well as the treatment process, and negotiate with the child some replacement behaviors given the behavioral function. The child's adherence with such guidance is not counted on in behavioral pediatrics, however, which is why the caregiver participates fully and is trained to serve as co-therapist. Selection of the functional communication response to train is based upon child and caregiver preferences with consideration of response effort and speed of acquisition as well as recognizability within the child's environment (see Houck, Dracobly, & Baak, 2023, for more guidance).

The caregiver can be directed by the clinician to remind the child each morning for a few days about the new skill to be displayed when needed, to train siblings as relevant, to prompt use of the skill as needed, and to engineer reinforcing responses when the skill is displayed. A reward program may also be devised and implemented for a time. Task analyses of many social skills pertaining to self-advocacy are found in Tierney and Green (2022).

Key Takeaways from this Chapter

- Another clinical metafactor to prioritize, as relevant, is poor self-advocacy skills, or failure to appropriately mand for attention, a break or some alone time, assistance, or a desired item. Children can be told by caregivers that they are allowed to disagree with those in authority but there is a right way and wrong way to do this, and be taught the difference.
- Teaching self-advocacy skills represents social skills training or mand training, and while children may be offered such instruction by the clinician directly, caregivers are always included in such endeavors to facilitate generalization and maintenance.

References

Costa, A., & Pelaez, M. (2014). Implementing intensive tact instruction to increase frequency of spontaneous mands and tacts in typically developing children. *Behavioral Development Bulletin, 19*, 19–24.

Drifke, M. A., Tiger, J. H., & Lillie, M. A. (2020). DRA contingencies promote improved tolerance to delayed reinforcement during FCT compared to DRO and fixed-time schedules. *Journal of Applied Behavior Analysis, 53*, 1579–1592.

Hanley, G. P., Heal, N. A., Tiger, J. H., & Ingvarsson, E. T. (2007). Evaluation of a classwide teaching program for developing preschool life skills. *Journal of Applied Behavior Analysis, 40*, 277–300.

Hixson, M. (2004). Behavioral cusps, basic behavioral repertoires, and cumulative-hierarchical learning. *Psychological Record, 54*, 387–403.

Houck, E. J., Dracobly, J. D., & Baak, S. A. (2023). A practitioner's guide for selecting functional communication responses. *Behavior Analysis in Practice, 16*, 65–75.

Tierney, J., & Green, E. (2022). *Teaching social skills to youth: An easy-to-follow guide to teaching 196 basic to complex life skills* (4th ed). Boys Town.

Tiger, J. H., Hanley, G. P., & Bruzek, J. (2008). Functional communication training: A review and practical guide. *Behavior Analysis in Practice, 1*, 16–23.

Other Clinical Problems **10**
Anxiety, Colic, Enuresis, Encopresis, and Habits and Tics

The preceding four chapters covered behavioral treatment of the clinical metafactors of sleep-related problems, behavioral noncompliance with caregiver directives, poor toleration of denial and delay, and poor self-advocacy skills. With those now shored up, we may proceed to a discussion of other clinical problems often encountered in behavioral pediatrics. Below, what works with childhood anxiety, excessive crying, enuresis, encopresis, toileting refusal, and habits and tics is discussed in abridged format. This section is by all means not comprehensive as that would go well beyond the scope of this book; the following sections are intended as a starting point for the practitioner who is hereby encouraged to review and incorporate additional sources of information and guidance.

Anxiety

Children report problems with anxiety more than anything else (Rapee *et al.*, 2022) and anxiety diagnoses are among the most common of all behavioral health diagnoses for children (Merikangas *et al.*, 2010). Not all cases of anxiety are clinically diagnosable and not all anxiety is harmful. We need at least some anxiety to care enough to study for that test tomorrow or to say the right things to our coworkers at challenging moments (cf. Yerkes & Dodson, 1908). It is therefore important for the practitioner, child, and family to know that anxiety, contrary to popular belief, is not the problem. Rather, avoidance of the circumstances that appear to the child to

DOI: 10.4324/9781003371281-11

trigger aversive thoughts, emotions, and bodily sensations is the problem. Here's why that is.

A large part of what we colloquially refer to as "anxiety" (i.e., sympathetic arousal) happens to be a critical part of evolved mammalian survival behavior. When risk is detected, the body enters survival mode, and this mode is uncomfortable. There is a mission-critical evolutionary advantage to this: what makes you feel this way within a threat-dense environment might kill or severely injure you, so it is to your advantage to feel that way and in turn to instinctually avoid what triggered it.

Yet the modern age is relatively bereft of encounters with apex predators and marauding malevolent tribes. Instead of lions and mortal enemies entering camp, those triggers for a typical present-day 6-year-old child include threats such as being left alone in bed in a dark room after lights-out. That aversive mental and bodily experience may nonetheless be similar, and attempting to avoid those triggering circumstances is human nature. It's *normal*, and these days simply a part of growing up.

For all anxiety-triggering circumstances that are unlikely to kill or severely injure, repeated exposure to the triggering circumstances serves to desensitize the risk detection circuitry, rendering the person wiser, braver, and more resilient to future such exposures. Anxious caregivers often fail to differentiate dangerous versus simply distressing circumstances, and will seek to remove any contact with triggering circumstances. This avoidance makes the child's short-term experience much more comfortable, but at the expense of opportunities to become wiser, braver, or more resilient. Anxiety is thus maintained via a negative reinforcement loop. It is no wonder that anxiety tends to worsen over time without effective treatment (Strauss *et al.*, 1988).

What works for anxiety is exposure. If the child is afraid of the dark, the child must be in the dark to overcome that fear. If the child is anxious about attending school, the child must attend school to overcome that anxiety. Of course, mere fear is not sufficient; the key is fear in the context of safety, to allow inhibitory learning to occur (e.g., Craske *et al.*, 2014). Thus, we want to ensure a safe overnight environment and a school environment conducive to learning before we embark upon exposure trials.

In some cases we will want to offer graduated exposure. Overcoming a fear of dogs may require a series of exposure opportunities, each successively involving the child and a gentle, well-trained dog coming physically closer to one another. Relaxation strategies such as diaphragmatic breathing, progressive muscle relaxation, grounding, visualization, and mediating responses such as "I can do this" are important to offer, but it must be asserted that these and other tools are intended to allow and facilitate more comfortable exposure and are not for the avoidance of anxiety.

My approach is to normalize the anxiety and the urge to avoid its triggers, ask the child what life would be like if the anxiety could right now be magically reduced, and explain that *we know how to help, but you have to trust me and the other adults in your life. The first few days will be challenging, but I believe in you. The key is to accept that feeling as normal, and live your life bravely anyway. It will soon get better, and you will be proud of yourself.* Assess for parenting, sibling dynamics, and classroom accommodations which facilitate experiential avoidance, and address them as needed. For worry, schedule a daily, 20-minute "Worry Time" at a time of day the child tends to not worry (and not within a couple hours of bedtime) and invite the child to share worries only at that time; otherwise, "It's not worry time, my dear."

Poor sleep is known to increase reactivity of the amygdala by more than 60% (Walker, 2017), so in cases of anxiety, it is important to assess for and address sleep problems and deficits. Hyperthyroidism and hypoglycemia are among the leading medical causes of anxiety in adults, and while relatively rare in children, acute and severe cases should be referred to the child's primary care physician for bloodwork at the physician's discretion.

While talking with the child about anxiety and steps to improve things can be helpful, it is usually resource-intensive and sometimes insufficient. Offering helpful conceptual and procedural guidance for caregivers can be very helpful given their potential influence on avoidance versus exposure experiences, and in fact a recent meta-analysis lends support for prescriptive behavioral treatment as a sole component in the treatment of childhood anxiety (Jewell, Wittkowski, & Pratt, 2022).

Colic

Excessive infant crying and inconsolability, also referred to as colic, has for decades been the most common concern for which medical advice is sought by caregivers during the child's first year of life, particularly within the first three months during which it is exhibited by up to 30% of infants (Forsyth, Leventhal, & McCarthy, 1985; Halpern & Coelho, 2016; Kaley, Reid, & Flynn, 2011). "Excessive crying" as a complaint may seem somewhat trivial to the physician or behavioral healthcare practitioner (especially those who have never experienced it as a parent) but, as a lived reality, it can severely impact maternal functioning and family life (Botha, Joronen, & Kaunonen,

2019; Oberklaid, 2000; Petzoldt, 2018), even years later (Halpern & Coelho, 2016; Rautava *et al.*, 1995).

Infant crying is normal and evolutionarily advantageous, as crying signals need and reliably elicits attention from caregivers (Soltis, 2004). Colic is generally thought to represent the extreme end of the normal crying continuum (Kaley, Reid, & Flynn, 2011; Oberklaid, 2000). Such extreme crying can (and understandably so) come to represent an unremitting aversive stimulus for caregivers. Maternal desperation and depression tend to result, particularly when the mother has a history of anxiety prior to pregnancy (Petzoldt, 2018). Impaired breastfeeding and family dynamics and increased possibility of abuse (e.g., shaken baby syndrome) are also known consequences (Botha, Joronen, & Kaunonen, 2019).

It is commonly believed by caregivers and professionals alike that excessive crying reflects an underlying medical condition such as constipation, gastroesophageal reflux, or food allergy, yet in reality this is very rarely the case (Barr, 2002; Oberklaid, 2000) and medication is generally not recommended (Halpern & Coelho, 2016). Management, alternatively, is implicated to a much greater degree, and this is the domain of the practitioner of behavioral pediatrics. The following are recommended for cases of excessive infant crying:

- Medical evaluation by the pediatrician before all else.
- Increase predictability for caregivers: If the infant is younger than 3 months old, inform the caregiver that chances are the crying will soon subside in frequency and intensity and that crying tends to cluster in the afternoon and evening for most infants (Oberklaid, 2000). Infants 6 to 8 weeks of age cry for an average total of 2 to 3 hours per 24 hours (with some crying for up to 6 hours; Royal Children's Hospital Melbourne, 2019) and may draw their legs up as if in pain; however, this is normal and not necessarily a sign of discomfort (sudden intense crying is a better indication of discomfort). It is also helpful for caregivers to hear that their job is to ensure the baby has what he or she needs, such as nourishment, clean diaper, a physically safe environment, and a sense of routine, and that this job description does not include keeping the child from crying. Crying *per se* is neither harmful nor an indication there is something wrong. Sometimes doing nothing is much more effective; trying too hard to stop the crying may serve to overstimulate the infant and prolong the crying (Ferber, 2006).
- When the infant is crying and the caregiver is reasonably certain the infant is safe and all needs are met (e.g., hunger, wet or soiled

diaper, pain), the caregiver is encouraged to leave the room during the crying and return to gently and lovingly interact when the crying tapers off (the caregiver may, however, approach the crying infant as the infant begins to cry to assess need). Besides demonstrating to the infant that social interaction is more likely when calm, letting the infant cry without attempting to soothe may facilitate onset of sleep, of which 2-month-olds require about 13.5 hours per 24 hours, with naps varying but becoming more regular and predictable by the third month of life, averaging 3 to 4 naps per day of about 1 to 1.5 hours each (Ferber, 2006). Differential attending may also serve to prevent future sleep problems otherwise stemming from the child learning to expect caregiver intervention facilitating sleep onset.

- Help the caregiver engineer a calm environment and establish consistent and predictable daily routines with respect to feeding, play, and sleep.
- Simulating the womb environment appears to help babies settle. Swaddling has been demonstrated to produce more self-regulatory ability, quietude, and sleep, and less arousal and physiological distress in infants; swaddling must however be discontinued when the infant begins to turn over from a supine to prone position which increases the risk of sudden infant death syndrome (van Sleuwen et al., 2007). Lester (2013) provides illustrated step-by-step guidance on how to swaddle the baby. Also, providing gentle, repetitive movement (i.e., while holding the baby and supporting the head and neck, offering slight and slow up-and-down movement) and simple, repetitive noise (e.g., white noise, metronome), and darkness or a dimly-lit environment can also help.
- Screen caregivers for anxiety and depression and offer relaxation strategies, supportive counseling, online resources, and/or referral to an appropriate behavioral healthcare provider as indicated (Long et al., 2018). Note that many caregivers who are anxious and/or depressed, particularly in cases in which onset came after the birth of the child, may benefit simply from an increased ability to predict the crying and knowledge that crying *per se* is a healthy activity for the baby. In the event daily peaks of crying are relatively predictable, suggest that the caregiver invite another trusted adult to take over for a few hours.
- The caregiver is encouraged to maintain a daily journal to record time of day, frequency, severity, and duration of crying, and intervention so that patterns may be discerned.

Enuresis

Enuresis is the name for bedwetting and daytime pants wetting. When the child has not yet been fully toilet trained, the term *primary enuresis* is used (up to 90% of all cases of enuresis are primary; Christophersen & Friman, 2010); otherwise, the term *secondary enuresis* is used. Enuresis is further subclassified based on when it occurs: *diurnal* is by day and *nocturnal* is by night (nocturnal enuresis is three to five times more common than diurnal; Shepard & Cox, 2017). Thus, a child who has been dry overnight but is now bedwetting is said to suffer from secondary nocturnal enuresis. Children under the age of 5 who wet are not diagnosed with enuresis; bedwetting and pants wetting are not atypical up to age 4 or so (Berk & Friman, 1990). About 20–25% of five-year-olds, 10% of ten-year-olds, and 3% of fifteen-year-olds wet the bed. About 6% of seven-year-olds wet by day (Christophersen & Vanscoyoc, 2013). Enuresis appears heritable (Christophersen & Friman, 2010) and is unlikely to involve psychiatric comorbidity (Friman *et al.*, 1998).

The clinician should collaborate with the child's primary care physician before treatment in order to rule out or address potential medical conditions such as urinary tract infection, constipation (which happens to be a powerful predictor of day wetting in particular; Loening-Baucke, 1997), urinary obstruction, diminished functional bladder capacity, diabetes, and others. The physician may refer the child on to a pediatric urologist for evaluation, in which case you will want to connect with that person as well.

The most effective and durable treatments for enuresis are behavior analytic in nature, with success rates reaching 90% (Mellon & McGrath, 2000; Ramakrishnan, 2008; Schroeder & Smith-Boydston, 2017). Christophersen and Friman (2010) offer a comprehensive review of behavioral treatments for enuresis including the urine alarm, retention control training, scheduled awakening, cleanliness training, overlearning, and use of rewards. They note that the urine alarm is known to be 65% to 80% effective over 5 to 12 weeks of use, with a six-month relapse rate of 15% to 30%. It may be used as the sole treatment component.

Schroeder and Smith-Boydston (2017) mention almost consistent use of the urine alarm across cases of nocturnal enuresis they treat, but I have found a high rate of success within two to three weeks (subsequent to addressing suboptimal clinical metafactors) with a behavioral treatment package rarely incorporating the alarm. This package typically includes the following:

- Medical evaluation by the pediatrician and/or pediatric urologist before all else.

- Removing all punishment and expressed disapproval.
- No more pull-ups.
- Clearly communicating expectations and increasing predictability. A supportive orientation meeting is held between parents and child before treatment commences during which the goal of becoming dry overnight and the planned procedures are discussed.
- Overlearning: Practicing the route from the bed to the potty multiple times in simulated conditions (i.e., just before lights-out, in pajamas, with all lights off except a bathroom nightlight, from being under the covers to sitting on the potty, and back to bed) with contingent praise.
- Scheduled awakening: The child is awakened just before the caregiver goes to bed, coinciding with what is likely to be the child's deepest sleep of the night (and if the child is already wet by then, the parent knows to wake the child a little earlier the next night). The caregiver gently ushers the half-awake child to the potty to urinate, then returns the child to bed with minimal social interaction. Considering the sleep literature along with that on enuresis, and that nocturnal enuresis is considered a parasomnia (Friman & Warzak, 1990), interrupting deep sleep prior to the occurrence of the parasomnia reduces the likelihood of the parasomnia – in this case, enuresis – for the remainder of the night (Meltzer & Crabtree, 2015). After a week of success, the caregiver skips a night, and further enuretic episodes prompt three more nights of waking followed by another skipped night. Note also that the most common cause of parasomnias is insufficient sleep (Meltzer & Crabtree, 2015), so ensure good sleep.
- Consequential effort: Cleanliness training. After the first three nights, if the child has wet the bed, the lights are turned on, the child is awakened and prompted to undress and help to place the wet clothing and bedding into the washing machine (to be run tomorrow), take a quick cool shower, get into clean pajamas, help the caregiver change the bedding (the change of clothing and bedding should be placed to the side ahead of time), and then return to bed. The caregiver is matter-of-fact and not emotional or talkative during this procedure.
- Contingent reinforcement: Dry nights are celebrated in the morning incorporating social and/or planned token reinforcement.
- Active collaboration: Caregiver knows to contact the clinician in the event of any questions or concerns.

The package described above tends to be successful with most young children but there will be cases that are more clinically complex and even seemingly intractable (i.e., "We've tried everything"). The practitioner should be prepared for such cases by reviewing the literature on enuresis, attending to clinical metafactor considerations, consulting interdisciplinary colleagues, and tailoring the treatment for the particular case while incorporating continuous measurement to ensure effectiveness. A solid history along with familiarity with the literature will offer clues previous clinicians have missed. For example, adenotonsillectomy may ultimately be indicated for some children with enuresis who snore heavily or show signs of sleep apnea; intriguingly, enuresis resolves immediately for about half of these children (American Psychiatric Association, 2022). Children presenting with intractable enuresis who also present with sleep-disordered breathing should be seen by a sleep specialist followed by pediatric otolaryngology, all in collaboration with the pediatrician.

Under the age of 5, especially when there is day wetting and bedwetting (these cases tend to arrive for services over the summer in anticipation of starting a new school), treatment may simply be educating caregivers on toilet training. Lastly, it should be noted that enuresis is one of the few "mental disorders" that ultimately resolves on its own, so treatment should be designed to compete and win against maturation effects.

Encopresis and Toileting Refusal

Encopresis is the name for defecation anywhere other than the toilet for children 4 years of age and older. Like enuresis, such cases are classified as primary or secondary, depending upon whether the child has ever been continent, with further subclassification into *retentive* (with constipation), constituting up to 95% of children referred for encopresis (Har & Croffie, 2010), and *nonretentive* (without constipation). Up to 7.5% of 6- to 12-year-olds experience encopresis, with the ratio of boys to girls as high as 6 to 1 (Har & Croffie, 2010; Schonwald & Rappaport, 2008). Encopresis itself does not predict psychiatric involvement (Friman et al., 1988). The vast majority of these children withhold stool (Partin et al., 1992) which is thought to be secondary to a history of painful bowel movements for most of these children, and therefore operant in nature; many children with a history of active avoidance of pain during the urge to defecate have developed paradoxical constriction of the external anal sphincter (Schroeder & Smith-Boydston, 2017). Healthy, regular defecation requires relaxation, not constriction, of that sphincter.

Encopresis is thus a good example of a clinical phenomenon at the nexus of medicine and behavior analysis, requiring collaboration between the practitioner of behavioral pediatrics and the child's pediatrician and/or pediatric gastroenterologist. Constipation in nearly all encopresis cases means a good chance of fecal impaction (71% chance, in fact; Partin *et al.*, 1992) and while a child is impacted (that is, the large intestine is so full of stool, the stool can't move on its own; this is colloquially referred to as a *blockage*), no progress with behavioral treatment is possible. Such medical conditions, including non-fecal obstruction, must therefore be identified and treated before behavioral treatment begins. Hirschsprung disease is a rarer condition that should be ruled out as well; this is a congenital disorder affecting intestinal motility and seen in four times as many boys as girls (Mahon & Khlevner, 2021). The majority of these cases are identified by the child's first birthday, but about 18% have not yet been diagnosed by age 4 (Loening-Baucke, 1994). Christophersen and Friman (2010) offer informative tables facilitating identification that may be used in developing your history questionnaire or intake interview for cases of encopresis, with red flags shared with the child's physician.

Behavioral treatment may commence once the large intestine, also referred to as the *bowel* or *colon*, has been entirely cleaned out (under the care of a physician) and a comprehensive history has been taken (see Christophersen & Friman, 2010, and Schroeder & Smith-Boydston, 2017, for excellent guidance regarding assessment). Active collaboration between behavior analyst and the child's physician will likely involve ongoing selection, titration, and facilitation of treatment adherence with the use of laxatives and stool softeners (e.g., MiraLAX) and supplemental fiber (e.g., Metamucil Thins) to maintain peristalsis and prevent a recurrence of constipation during a course of behavioral treatment. Relatedly, caregivers should be told how diarrhea or fecal smudging in the underwear may in fact represent seepage around a fecal mass from a recurrence of constipation following clean out – a condition for which the last thing we would want to do is treat with over-the-counter (OTC) antidiarrheal medications (Christophersen & Friman, 2010).

The following represent components of an effective course of treatment which may be successful in as little as six weeks (e.g., Stark *et al.*, 1997), but may take up to a year (Schroeder & Smith-Boydston, 2017) for independent defecation on the toilet without the need for OTC medications. The meta-factor of noncompliance, if present, may have to be addressed before treatment for encopresis will be successful (McMahon & Forehand, 2003).

• Effective directive delivery, such as directing, not requesting, that the child visit the toilet. It may take several months for the recently evacuated large intestine to heal and for children to begin perceiving the urge to defecate, which is why encopretic children shouldn't be asked whether they have to go

- Dietary changes: more fiber and fluid intake (i.e., water and fruit juices), and less milk, cheese, and refined sugar
- Sufficient daily exercise to trigger the orthocolic reflex
- Regularly scheduled mealtimes
- Regularly scheduled potty sits
- Provision of a stepstool in front of the toilet for proper foot positioning and leverage
- Differential attending and an incentivization system tied to all desired relevant behavior and clean pants-checks
- A letter to the school requesting a more private restroom, and fruit juice in place of milk
- Avoidance of medications with which constipation is a side effect

Guidelines for toilet-sit scheduling generally call for a daily 5- to 10-minute sit about 20 minutes following the meal closest to the time the child lately tends to move his or her bowels. This is most commonly after school (Levine, 1976), so for most, dinnertime it is. All punishment attempts related to toileting should be eliminated, and visiting the toilet should be rewarded in various ways. I routinely recommend allowing electronic tablet use (if the family has already introduced this infernal device) only while seated on the potty during the course of treatment; an alternative is for caregivers to sit on the side of the bathtub and hang out or read with the child. Otherwise, having to sit on the potty may be perceived by the child as an unearned time-out, which increases the likelihood of toileting avoidance.

Nonretentive encopresis constitutes around 5% of all cases of encopresis, and these cases tend to be relatively more clinically complex. Consideration of and addressing relevant clinical metafactors may be critical for success, as would be addressing toileting skills.

Another group comprises preschool-age children, usually presenting with no other behavioral concerns, who regularly and happily produce bowel movements in their pants but refuse to use the toilet for defecation. This group may be as large as 22% of all 3- to 5-year-olds (Taubman, 1997). Regular bowel movements suggest little need for initial medical evaluation, although obtaining a good history remains critically important. Christophersen and Friman (2010) offer a treatment method involving the shaping of potty pooping, going from the child defecating in the pull-up while standing in the bathroom, to sitting on the potty while wearing the pull-up and defecating in the pull-up, to defecating on the toilet without the pull-up, with any number of intermediate steps. I have found a fear of being splashed by toilet water to be partly behind potty refusal in one recent case; turning off the fill valve and gradually allowing more water to fill the bowl after each flush turned out to be a necessary component. Successive approximations are reinforced, with the most salient rewards delivered contingently upon the final step or two of each trial. Proactive consideration of diet, exercise, and behavioral compliance is also recommended.

Habits and Tics

Habits such as thumb sucking, hair pulling or twirling, nail biting, cheek chewing, lip biting, skin picking, and pencil tapping are persistent, repetitive, largely mindless behaviors. Approximately a third to half of preschool children engage in thumb sucking, for example, which disappears in all but 5% to 15% by age 5 (Blenner, 2019). Many other habits are common for children and adults (Miltenberger, Fuqua, & Woods, 1998). The line between "normal" and "worthy of intervention" is drawn where such habits cause physical harm or otherwise interfere with development and functioning (Schroeder & Smith-Boydston, 2017). Generally, however, habits are not treated before the age of 4 except with the use of differential attending (Christophersen & Vanscoyoc, 2013).

Tics are sudden repetitive motor movements or vocalizations (e.g., uttering words, clearing the throat, or making barking sounds) that represent "isolated disinhibited fragments of normal motor or vocal behaviors" (Leckman, King, & Cohen, 1999). About a quarter of all children exhibit a tic of short duration at some point in their childhood. Chronic tics – those lasting for over a year – are seen in only 1% of children, and Tourette syndrome, the diagnosis of which requires longstanding multiple motor tics and at least one vocal tic, is far more rare (Peterson, Campise, & Azrin, 1994). The median onset of tics appears to be age 5 or 6, with greatest tic severity occurring between ages 7 and 15 (Leckman et al., 1999).

The vast majority of those with tics report premonitory sensations and urges. The experience of having tics tends to be described as an oncoming sneeze; it's much easier and more satisfying to sneeze than to stifle. These urges can be experienced as worse than the tics themselves (Woods et al., 2008). As discussed by Miltenberger and colleagues (2020), those aversive physical and mental premonitory sensations and urges may be seen as establishing operations, and they appear to ebb once the habit or tic is exhibited. This is automatic negative reinforcement at work. This does not capture all cases but it may represent most; habits and tics may also be maintained by positive reinforcement (social or sensory) or even representative of adjunctive behavior (Miltenberger, Fuqua, & Woods, 1998; Wagaman, Miltenberger, & Williams, 1995). And, "nervous habits" are not necessarily due to being nervous, as Woods and Miltenberger (1996) found.

Successful treatment of simple habits can be relatively straightforward. Treatment of thumb sucking, for example, generally involves differential attending and application of a commercially available aversive-tasting solution to the thumb (Friman, Barone, & Christophersen, 1986). A reward contingency may be added (Friman & Leibowitz, 1990). Interestingly, when a habit tends to co-occur with another habit (termed *habit covariance*), directly treating one may successfully indirectly treat the other. For example, when thumb sucking and hair pulling covary, treatment of thumb sucking tends to reduce or eliminate the hair pulling as well (Friman & Hove, 1987; Watson & Allen, 1993). Linus gave up his blue blanket this way (Friman, 1990).

More is needed for other, more complex habits and tics. Helping professionals struggled for decades to help to little avail. Then along came Azrin and Nunn (1973) with a shocking announcement:

> No clinical treatment for nervous habits has been generally effective. … A new procedure was devised for counteracting these influences … The treatment was given during a single session to 12 clients who had diverse nervous habits such as nail-biting, thumb-sucking, eyelash-picking, head-jerking, shoulder-jerking, tongue-pushing and lisping. The habits were virtually eliminated on the very first day for all 12 clients and did not return during the extended follow-up for the 11 clients who followed the instructions.
>
> (p. 619)

This new procedure, appearing a few years later in their mass-market book *Habit Control in a Day* (Azrin & Nunn, 1977) and purported to have a 99.5% success rate with over 300 clients, was called *habit reversal training* (HRT). Originally consisting of a package of 13 treatment components, subsequent research has winnowed this down to only three or four components. The resulting treatment package has been referred to as abbreviated or simplified HRT (Jones, Swearer, & Friman, 1997; Miltenberger, Fuqua, & Woods, 1998) and generally involves 1) awareness training, 2) the selection and practice of replacement behaviors that when practiced render the habit or tic momentarily motorically unpracticable (see Woods *et al.*, 2008, pp. 45–46, for a wonderfully helpful list of potential replacement behaviors by tic topography), 3) social support (e.g., prompting, delivering contingent reinforcement), and 4) when the habit or tic appears to be associated with anxiety, relaxation training.

The eventual application of functional analysis methodology to the assessment and treatment of habits and tics proved advantageous (e.g., Rapp et al., 1999; Watson & Sterling, 1998). Extending this line of applied research, Woods, Piacentini, and their colleagues (Piacentini et al., 2010; Woods et al., 2008) updated the modern HRT package by applying function-based components while reintroducing some original HRT components, labeling this new package *comprehensive behavioral intervention for tics* (CBIT). The CBIT package, manualized for practitioners (Woods et al., 2008) and put to the test via randomized controlled trial (Piacentini et al., 2010), includes simplified HRT plus inconvenience review, contingency management, and relapse prevention programming.

Some treatment considerations for habits and tics include the following:

- HRT is quite effective without function-based assessment and treatment components, but some cases may require them. Habits and tics appear operant in nature.
- Research does not support the lore that when children intentionally suppress their tics at school, they experience a tic explosion when they get home (Woods et al., 2008). The after-school tic explosion appears to be more due to the influence of setting events than to active suppression. Extinction of contingent attention, for example, may be an important treatment component (see, for example, Watson & Sterling, 1988).
- Contingent social and token reinforcement for absence of tics and habits, and response cost contingent upon occurrence, have been shown to be helpful (see Miltenberger et al., 2020, for discussion).
- When two simple habits covary, consider directly treating one in order to indirectly treat the other.
- Replacement behaviors for tics do not necessarily need to be incompatible with the tic (Sharenow, Fuqua, & Miltenberger, 1989; Woods et al., 1999) but should nonetheless be compatible with activities of daily life (Woods et al., 2010).
- The use of technology may be helpful in increasing awareness for habits and tics (Himle et al., 2018; Rapp, Miltenberger, & Long, 1998).
- While supportive talk therapy can be a helpful component in the comprehensive treatment of habits and tics, talk therapy alone is ineffective (Kyoung et al., 2021).

Key Takeaways from this Chapter

• Childhood anxiety is common, as is well-intended caregiver accommodation resulting in negatively reinforced avoidance habits (for all parties). Children and caregivers require guidance as to how negative reinforcement serves to maintain anxiety, and how repeated exposure to (non-dangerous) feared stimuli offers desensitization and inhibitory learning. Relaxation strategies may also be taught, but with emphasis on their function – not for the avoidance of anxiety, but to increase willingness to engage in exposure trials. Worry Time is a means of offering exposure for the child and improving treatment adherence of the caregiver. Ensuring physical health and good sleep are important in the assessment and treatment of anxiety.

• Excessive crying, or colic, represents the extreme end of the normal crying continuum and severely impacts maternal functioning and family life sometimes leading to physical abuse. It is the most common reason for seeking medical advice during the first year of a child's life. Despite common lore, colic is rarely due to an underlying medical condition such as constipation, gastroesophageal reflux, or food allergy. Crying is not necessarily an indication that something is wrong, particularly when the baby has been fed, has a clean diaper, is in a safe environment, and is in a routine.

• Enuresis is the name for bedwetting and daytime pants wetting that have no known medical cause for children 5 years of age and older. Medical rule-outs come before behavioral treatment. Behavioral treatment is usually successful and involves some combination of the urine alarm, retention control training, stream interruption exercises, scheduled awakening, overlearning, cleanliness training, and use of rewards, if not the urine alarm alone. Enuresis will eventually resolve on its own but we need not wait given effective treatment available.

• Encopresis is the name for defecation anywhere other than the toilet for children 4 years of age and older. The vast majority of encopretic cases involve withholding stool, constipation, and fecal impaction, and many of these cases are thought to involve the development of paradoxical constriction of the external anal sphincter from a history of active avoidance of painful bowel movements. Successful treatment of encopresis with constipation requires active collaboration between the clinician and the child's pediatrician and/or gastroenterologist.

• Habits (e.g., thumb sucking, nail biting) and tics (e.g., shoulder shrugging, throat clearing) are repetitive behaviors occurring outside of full awareness or intention. Simple habits like thumb sucking may be successfully treated using differential attending, a mildly aversive consequence for engagement (e.g., aversive-tasting solution on the thumb), and a reward contingency. Otherwise, HRT, and its latest iteration, CBIT, enjoy empirical support, as do contingent social and token reinforcement for absence of tics and habits with response cost contingent upon their occurrence.

References

American Psychiatric Association (2022). *Diagnostic and statistical manual of mental disorders* (5th ed., text rev.). Author.

Azrin, N. H., & Nunn, R. G. (1973). Habit-reversal: A method of eliminating nervous habits and tics. *Behaviour Research and Therapy, 11,* 619–628.

Azrin, N. H., & Nunn, R. G. (1977). *Habit control in a day.* Simon and Schuster.

Barr, R. G. (2002). Changing our understanding of infant colic. *Archives of Pediatric and Adolescent Medicine, 156,* 1172–1174.

Berk, L. B., & Friman, P. C. (1990). Epidemiological aspects of toilet training. *Clinical Pediatrics, 29,* 278–282.

Blenner, S. (2019). Thumb-sucking. In M. Augustyn & B. Zuckerman (Eds.), *Zuckerman Parker handbook of developmental and behavioral pediatrics for primary care* (4th ed., pp. 424–426). Wolters Kluwer.

Botha, E., Joronen, K., & Kaunonen, M. (2019). The consequences of having an excessively crying infant in the family: An integrative literature review. *Scandinavian Journal of Caring Sciences, 33,* 779–790.

Christophersen, E. R., & Friman, P. C. (2010). *Elimination disorders in children and adolescents.* Hogrefe.

Christophersen, E. R., & Vanscoyoc, S. M. (2013). *Treatments that work with children: Empirically supported strategies for managing childhood problems* (2nd ed.). American Psychological Association.

Craske, M. G., Treanor, M., Conway, C. C., Zbozinek, T., & Vervliet, B. (2014). Maximizing exposure therapy: An inhibitory learning approach. *Behaviour Research and Therapy, 58,* 10–23.

Ferber, R. (2006). *Solve your child's sleep problems (rev. ed.).* Fireside.

Forsyth, B. W., Leventhal, J. M., & McCarthy, P. L. (1985). Mothers' perceptions of problems of feeding and crying behaviors: A prospective study. *The American Journal of Diseases of Children, 139,* 269–272.

Friman, P. C. (1990). Concurrent habits: What would Linus do with his blanket if his thumb-sucking were treated? *American Journal of Diseases of Children, 144,* 1316–1318.

Friman, P. C., Barone, V. J., & Christophersen, E. R. (1986). Aversive taste treatment of finger and thumb sucking. *Pediatrics, 78,* 174–176.

Friman, P. C., Handwerk, M. L., Swearer, S. M., McGinnis, J. C., & Warzak, W. J. (1998). Do children with primary nocturnal enuresis have clinically significant behavior problems? *Archives of Pediatrics and Adolescent Medicine, 152,* 537–539.

Friman, P. C., & Hove, G. (1987). Apparent covariation between child habit disorders: Effects of successful treatment for thumb sucking on untargeted chronic hair pulling. *Journal of Applied Behavior Analysis, 20,* 421–425.

Friman, P. C., & Leibowitz, J. M. (1990). An effective and acceptable treatment alternative for chronic thumb- and finger-sucking. *Journal of Pediatric Psychology, 15,* 57–65.

Friman, P. C., Mathews, J. R., Finney, J. W., Christophersen, E. R., & Leibowitz, J. M. (1988). Do encopretic children have clinically significant behavior problems? *Pediatrics, 82,* 407–409.

Friman, P. C., & Warzak, W. J. (1990). Nocturnal enuresis: A prevalent, persistent, yet curable parasomnia. *Pediatrician, 17,* 38–45.

Halpern, R., & Coelho, R. (2016). Excessive crying in infants. *Jornal de Pediatria, 92,* S40–S45.

Har, A. F., & Croffie, J. M. (2010). Encopresis. *Pediatrics in Review, 31,* 368–374.

Himle, J. A., Bybee, D., O'Donnell, L. A., Weaver, A., Vlnka, S., DeSena, D. T., & Rimer, J. M. (2018). Awareness enhancing and monitoring device plus habit reversal in the treatment of trichotillomania: An open feasibility trial. *Journal of Obsessive-Compulsive and Related Disorders, 16,* 14–20.

Jewell, C., Wittkowski, A., & Pratt, D. (2022). The impact of parent-only interventions on child anxiety: A systematic review and meta-analysis. *Journal of Affective Disorders, 309,* 324–349.

Jones, K. M., Swearer, S. M., & Friman, P. C. (1997). Relax and try this instead: Abbreviated habit reversal for maladaptive self-biting. *Journal of Applied Behavior Analysis, 30,* 697–699.

Kaley, F., Reid, V., & Flynn, E. (2011). The psychology of infant colic: A review of current research. *Infant Mental Health Journal, 32,* 526–541.

Kyoung, M. K., Bae, E., Lee, J., Park, T. W., & Myung, H. L. (2021). A review of cognitive and behavioral interventions for tic disorder. *Journal of the Korean Academy of Child and Adolescent Psychiatry, 32,* 51–62.

Leckman, J. F., King, R. A., & Cohen, D. J. (1999). Tics and tic disorders. In J. F. Leckman & D. J. Cohen (Eds.), *Tourette's syndrome: Developmental psychopathology and clinical care* (pp. 23–42). Wiley.

Lester, J. (2013). *Survivor's guide to colic.* Green Jester.

Levine, M. D. (1976). Children with encopresis: A study of treatment outcome. *Pediatrics, 56,* 845–852.

Loening-Baucke, V. A. (1994). Management of chronic constipation in infants and toddlers. *American Family Physician, 49,* 397–400, 403–406, 411–413.

Loening-Baucke, V. (1997). Urinary incontinence and urinary tract infection and their resolution with treatment of chronic constipation of childhood. *Pediatrics, 100,* 228–232.

Long, J., Powell, C., Bamber, D., Garratt, R., Brown, J., Dyson, S., & St. James-Roberts, I. (2018). Development of materials to support parents whose babies cry excessively: Findings and health service implications. *Primary Health Care Research and Development, 19,* 320–332.

Mahon, M., & Khlevner, J. (2021). Hirschsprung disease. *Pediatrics in Review, 42,* 714–716.

McMahon, R. J., & Forehand, R. L. (2003). *Helping the noncompliant child: Family-based treatment for oppositional behavior* (2nd ed.). Guilford.

Mellon, M. W., & McGrath, M. L. (2000). Empirically supported treatments in pediatric psychology: Nocturnal enuresis. *Journal of Pediatric Psychology, 25*, 193–214.

Meltzer, L., & Crabtree, V. (2015). *Pediatric sleep problems: A clinician's guide to behavioral interventions.* American Psychological Association.

Merikangas, K. R., He, J., Burstein, M., Swanson, S. A., Avenevoli, S., Cui, L., Benjet, C., Georgiades, K., & Swendsen, J. (2010). Lifetime prevalence of mental disorders in US adolescents: Results from the national comorbidity study-adolescent supplement (NCS-A). *Journal of the American Academy of Child and Adolescent Psychiatry, 49*, 980–989.

Miltenberger, R. G., Fuqua, R. W., & Woods, D. W. (1998). Applying behavior analysis to clinical problems: Review and analysis of habit reversal. *Journal of Applied Behavior Analysis, 31*, 447–469.

Miltenberger, R. G., Stiede, J. T., Woods, D. W., & Himle, M. B. (2020). Tic disorders and trichotillomania. In P. Sturmey (Ed.), *Functional analysis in clinical treatment* (2nd ed., pp. 177–198). Academic.

Oberklaid, F. (2000). Persistent crying in infancy: A persistent clinical conundrum. *Journal of Paediatrics and Child Health, 36*, 297–298.

Partin, J. C., Hamill, S. K., Fischel, J. E., & Partin, J. S. (1992). Painful defecation and fecal soiling in children. *Pediatrics, 89*, 1007–1009.

Peterson, A. L., Campise, R. L., & Azrin, N. H. (1994). Behavioral and pharmacological treatments for tic and habit disorders: A review. *Developmental and Behavioral Pediatrics, 15*, 430–441.

Petzoldt, J. (2018). Systematic review on maternal depression versus anxiety in relation to excessive infant crying: It is all about the timing. *Archives of Women's Mental Health, 21*, 15–30.

Piacentini, J., Woods, D. W., Scahill, L., Wilhelm, S., Peterson, A. L., Chang, S., Ginsberg, G. S., Deckersbach, T., Dziura, J., Levi-Pearl, S., & Walkup, J. T. (2010). Behavior therapy for children with tourette disorder: A randomized controlled trial. *JAMA: The Journal of the American Medical Association, 303*, 1929–1937.

Ramakrishnan, K. (2008). Evaluation and treatment of enuresis. *American Family Physician, 78*, 489–496.

Rapee, R., Wignail, A., Spence, S., Cobham, V., & Lyneham, H. (2022). *Helping your anxious child: A step-by-step guide for parents* (3rd ed.). New Harbinger.

Rapp, J. T., Miltenberger, R. G., Galensky, T. L., Ellingson, S. A., & Long, E. S. (1999). A functional analysis of hair pulling. *Journal of Applied Behavior Analysis, 32*, 329–337.

Rapp, J. T., Miltenberger, R. G., & Long, E. S. (1998). Augmenting simplified habit reversal with an awareness enhancement device: Preliminary findings. *Journal of Applied Behavior Analysis, 31*, 665–668.

Rautava, P., Lehtonen, L., Helenius, H., & Sillanpaa, M. (1995). Infantile colic: Child and family three years later. *Pediatrics, 96*, 43–47.

Royal Children's Hospital Melbourne (2019). *Unsettled or crying babies.* Author. www.rch.org.au/clinicalguide/guideline_index/Crying_Baby_Infant_Distress/

Schonwald, A. D., & Rappaport, L. A. (2008). Elimination conditions. In M. L. Wolraich, D. D. Drotar, P. H. Dworkin, & E. C. Perrin (Eds.), *Developmental-behavioral pediatrics* (pp. 791–804). Mosby.

Schroeder, C. S., & Smith-Boydston, J. M. (2017). *Assessment and treatment of childhood problems: A clinician's guide* (3rd ed.). Guilford.

Sharenow, E. L., Fuqua, R. W., & Miltenberger, R. G. (1989). The treatment of muscle tics with dissimilar competing response practice. *Journal of Applied Behavior Analysis, 22*, 35–42.

Shepard, J. A., & Cox, D. J. (2017). Elimination disorders: Enuresis and encopresis. In M. C. Roberts & R. G. Steele (Eds.), *Handbook of pediatric psychology* (5th ed.), pp. 442–451.

Soltis, J. (2004). The signal functions of early infant crying. *Behavioral and Brain Sciences, 27*, 443–458.

Stark, L. J., Opipari, L. C., Donaldson, D. L., Danovsky, M. B., Rasile, D. A., & DelSanto, A. F. (1997). Evaluation of a standard protocol for retentive encopresis: A replication. *Journal of Pediatric Psychology, 22*, 619–633.

Strauss, C., Lease, C., Last, C., & Francis, G. (1988). Overanxious disorder: An examination of developmental differences. *Journal of Abnormal Child Psychology, 11*, 433–443.

Taubman, B. (1997). Toilet training and toileting refusal for stool only: A prospective study. *Pediatrics, 99*, 54–58.

van Sleuwen, B. E., Engelbarts, A. C., Boere-Boonekamp, M. M., Kuis, W., Schulpen, T. W. J., & L'Hoir, M. P. (2007). Swaddling: A systematic review. *Pediatrics, 120*, e1097–e1106. 10.1542/peds.2006-2083

Wagaman, J. R., Miltenberger, R. G., & Williams, D. E. (1995). Treatment of a vocal tic by differential reinforcement. *Journal of Behavior Therapy and Experimental Psychiatry, 26*, 35–39.

Walker, M. (2017). *Why we sleep: Unlocking the power of sleep and dreams.* Scribner.

Watson, T. S., & Allen, K. D. (1993). Elimination of thumb sucking as a treatment for severe trichotillomania. *Journal of the American Academy of Child and Adolescent Psychiatry, 32*, 830–834.

Watson, T. S., & Sterling, H. E. (1998). Brief functional analysis and treatment of a vocal tic. *Journal of Applied Behavior Analysis, 31*, 471–474.

Woods, D. W., & Miltenberger, R. G. (1996). Are persons with nervous habits nervous? A preliminary examination of habit function in a nonreferred population. *Journal of Applied Behavior Analysis, 29*, 259–261.

Woods, D. W., Murray, L. K., Fuqua, R. W., Seif, T. A., Boyer, L. J., & Siah, A. (1999). Comparing the effectiveness of similar and dissimilar competing responses in evaluating the habit reversal treatment for oral-digital habits in children. *Journal of Behavior Therapy and Experimental Psychiatry, 30*, 289–300.

Woods, D. W., Piacentini, J. C., Chang, S. W., Deckersbach, T., Ginsberg, G. S., Peterson, A. L., Scahill, L. D., Walkup, J. T., & Wilhelm, S. (2008). *Managing Tourette syndrome: A behavioral intervention for children and adults.* Oxford.

Yerkes, R. M., & Dodson, J. D. (1908). The relation of strength of stimulus to rapidity of habit-formation. *Journal of Comparative Neurology and Psychology, 18*, 459–482.

Caregiver Treatment Adherence   **11**

Treatment effectiveness, efficiency, and durability in behavioral pediatrics rely heavily on success with prescriptive behavioral treatment, itself requiring caregivers' consistent follow-through with recommended procedures. This follow-through by caregivers is what we call *treatment adherence*, and its importance is impossible to overstate. Treatment *compliance* and *adherence* are synonymous (Watson, Foster, & Friman, 2006) with "adherence" the preferred term (Rapoff, 2010) so as to reflect multivariate causality and to avoid verbally framing the client or caregiver as to blame (Stimson, 1974). A related term, treatment *fidelity*, refers to the extent to which the treatment is delivered by the clinician as designed. Caregiver adherence with treatment recommendations is the focus of this chapter.

Problems with treatment adherence put treatment effectiveness at risk, slow progress, prolong suffering, and increase behavioral healthcare utilization and costs. Because nonadherence is predicted in about 20% to 50% of families receiving behavioral health services that require caregiver follow-through (Kazdin, 1996; Moore & Simons, 2011) and clinicians tend to overestimate adherence rates (Varni, 1983), it is critically important for clinicians to anticipate nonadherence and to be familiar with factors predicting it. It is not *whether* it will occur but *to what extent*, and clinicians should work to proactively minimize and reactively improve it.

Medical nonadherence for adults hovers around 50%, but adherence improves with greater lethality and pain associated with the medical condition; the highest adherence rates are associated with cancer and arthritis, whereas the lowest are associated with pulmonary disease, diabetes, and

DOI: 10.4324/9781003371281-12

sleep problems (DiMatteo, 2004). Unanticipated side effects are also associated with lower adherence (Levensky & O'Donohue, 2006). Although some early data exist to suggest caregiver adherence with medical regimens for their children, while low, is still higher than for themselves (Maatar & Yaffe, 1974), caregivers' adherence with behavioral health regimens for their children can be more challenging, and thus worse given a host of other variables such as child noncompliance, developmental factors, and the negative influence of other family members (Moore & Amado, 2021; Rapoff, 2010). Treatments of longer duration and higher cost, and treatments which interfere with caregiver lifestyle, are associated with lower adherence (Levensky & O'Donohue, 2006; Varni, 1983).

Maintaining high treatment adherence is likely to be more challenging when the child is older (Target & Fonagy, 2005) and the problem has been longstanding (Levensky & O'Donohue, 2006; Varni, 1983). Caregivers are more likely to follow through with clinician directives when their children are more likely to follow through with their directives (Watson, Foster, & Friman, 2006). Notably, *moderate* problem severity appears to predict the greatest adherence in behavioral health; lower adherence is predicted when the problem behavior is not serious enough to threaten health or daily activity (Levensky & O'Donohue, 2006; Varni, 1983) but also when it is much more severe (Stocco & Thompson, 2015) and complex (Target & Fonagy, 2005).

Problems with treatment adherence are more likely when the caregiver is a single parent, is less educated, or when there is socioeconomic disadvantage (Allen & Warzak, 2000; Target & Fonagy, 2005). However, such sociodemographic variables alone are not predictive of nonadherence but a combination of these along with more below *are* predictive (Varni, 1983). Caregivers with a history of ADHD, antisocial behavior, substance overuse, depression, and insecurity of attachment are more likely to be nonadherent with treatment recommendations (Target & Fonagy, 2005), as are those with interfering health problems such as memory or visual challenges (Levensky & O'Donohue, 2006) or other cognitive impairment that hurt their ability to comprehend their responsibilities (Allen & Warzak, 2000). Stressful life events, marital discord, and social isolation, and low social support also predict nonadherence (Allen & Warzak, 2000; Stocco & Thompson, 2015; Target & Fonagy, 2005). One versus both parents attending appointments is also predictive of lower adherence, as are situations in which caregivers did not seek the treatment as in cases of mandated attendance, or when they otherwise perceive a lack of need for treatment (Target & Fonagy, 2005). All of these factors have the potential to impact caregivers' ability to control and alter their home environment to facilitate adherence (Sanders & Glynn, 1981).

A number of models for understanding and addressing nonadherence have been developed through the years but only behavior-analytic models have shown effectiveness (Moore & Amado, 2021), a likely reflection of the use of contingency analysis, which also lends to the 90%-plus effectiveness rate of behavioral interventions (Fisher *et al.*, 2023). Caregiver adherence to treatment recommendations, after all, is an operant class and a form of generalized responding (Moore & Amado, 2021; Stokes & Baer, 1977), and treatment recommendations are likely to be in competition with the previously existing contingencies that maintained unhelpful parenting strategies (Allen & Warzak, 2000). Indeed, parenting behavior is a product of historical and current circumstances including those pertaining to child behavior (Stocco & Thompson, 2015); child behavior, among other factors, naturally shapes and maintains caregiver behavior. Stocco and Thompson (2015) refer to Patterson's (1976) concept of the *negative reinforcement trap* and Wahler's (1976) concept of the *positive reinforcement trap*; the former involves relief for the caregiver via avoidance of or giving in to extinction bursts, and the latter involves, for example, spending quality time with a young child avoiding school by pretending to be ill; in each case, the caregiver's immediate experience is improved but the wrong message is being sent to the child.

Assessment of Treatment Adherence

Caregiver treatment adherence may be assessed via caregiver self-report and self-monitoring, blood work (in cases of medication or diet adherence, for example), video recording, or direct observation of implementation (Levensky & O'Donohue, 2006; McNeil & Hembree-Kigin, 2010; Rapoff, 2010; Varni, 1983). Everything relevant to adherence, or, perhaps only those variables critical to client health or most associated with aversiveness for caregivers may be selected for measurement. And some measures may be more reliable than others; for example, pill counts do not necessarily reflect how many have been ingested (Friman, 2021a). Note also that continuous measurement of treatment effects may be viewed as a reasonable proxy for the continuous measurement of adherence. If data trends are flat, either the wrong treatment was selected, the caregiver was inadequately trained in the procedures to implement, or the procedures are simply not being implemented.

Adherence-associated behaviors also may be functionally analyzed. Allen and Warzak (2000) urged behavior analysts to "look beyond the contingencies that control the behavior of the child and to look at those that control the behavior of the parent. It is these contingencies that determine parental adherence" (p. 387). Functional behavior assessment, reviewed in Chapter 3, may be used for this purpose (Watson, Foster, & Friman, 2006).

Simply measuring adherence can impact it (Friman, 2021a). This phenomenon is leveraged in business (e.g., "employees do what you review"); it may also be leveraged in behavioral pediatrics.

Programming for High Caregiver Treatment Adherence

Clinicians must beware of the fundamental attribution error; technically, nonadherence does not reflect caregiver laziness or absentmindedness but may reflect the clinician's failure to anticipate or address it effectively (Friman, 2021a). The immediate circumstances are more influential on performance than overall history (Lattal & Neef, 1996), so caregivers must be given direction as to how to engineer their environment to facilitate adherence, and rules to follow for challenging moments (Stocco & Thompson, 2015).

Strategies for improving treatment adherence involve rapport building, collaboration in treatment design, features of the treatment itself, caregiver education and training, and the antecedents and consequences of adherent behavior. These are discussed below.

Rapport

Caregivers demonstrably prefer empathy and interpersonal warmth over effective treatment (Chadwell *et al.*, 2019), so "soft skills" are critical for both high treatment adherence and clinical success (Rohrer *et al.*, 2021). Carl Rogers' (1957) necessary and sufficient conditions for therapeutic success famously included unconditional positive regard and an accurate, empathic understanding of the client's (and, with *our* caseload, the caregiver's) perspective. Clinicians may also use appropriate self-disclosure and humor (Shriver & Allen, 2008) and ensure that staff are friendly and helpful (Levensky & O'Donohue, 2006; Varni, 1983).

A longstanding recommendation for rapport building and maintaining high treatment acceptability and adherence has been to avoid or be judicious in using the technical language of behavior analysis (Allen, Barone, & Kuhn,

1993; Allen & Warzak, 2000; Baer, Wolf, & Risley, 1987; Bailey, 1991; Bailey & Burch, 2010; Becirevic, Critchfield, & Reed, 2016; Critchfield *et al.*, 2017; Foxx, 1996; Friman, 2014, 2017, 2021b; Lindsley, 1991; Rolider & Axelrod, 2005; Shriver & Allen, 2008; St. Peter, Pence, & Kestner, 2017). Our technical jargon has been characterized as a distinct dialect of English (Hineline, 1980) foreign to those we serve and with whom we collaborate. Importantly, however, context appears to play a role (Normand & Donohue, 2022); the use of technical language does not appear to degrade treatment acceptability when context is provided. Perhaps best practice would be to simply employ language comprehensible to the listener and use jargon only when doing so would make the message clearer. For instance, while I generally avoid the use of technical language, there are times when it is beneficial to communicate that engineering principles are at play. The concepts and implications of negative reinforcement and the extinction burst are discussed but are then translated to "relief as reward" and "shaking the vending machine," respectively.

While clinician behavior is important, caregiver nonadherence with prescribed behavioral treatment also requires remembering to do it (Jones *et al.*, 2021; also see Chacko *et al.*, 2009; Chacko *et al.*, 2013; and Nock & Kazdin, 2005). Caregivers, "like everyone else," noted Allen and Warzak (2000), "will most often engage in behavior that results in (a) more frequent reinforcement, (b), a greater magnitude of reinforcement, (c), more immediate reinforcement, and (d) less response effort" (p. 383), and so it is important to help the caregiver program and post prompts and for the clinician to be established as a conditioned reinforcer that maintains working for temporally distant rewards.

Collaboration

Caregivers benefit from a collaborative process (Levensky & O'Donohue, 2006; Shriver & Allen, 2008) including collaborative goal setting and selection of outcome measures (Cohrs *et al.*, 2016; Levensky & O'Donohue, 2006; Watson, Foster, & Friman, 2006). The process should be tailored for goodness of fit with the caregiver's lifestyle and natural sources of reinforcement (Levensky & O'Donohue, 2006). Greater treatment adherence is also associated with clinician accessibility, so clinicians should welcome frequent contact (Levensky & O'Donohue, 2006; Shriver & Allen, 2008; Watson, Foster, & Friman, 2006), minimize barriers to scheduling (Levensky & O'Donohue, 2006), and allow client families to stay with the same clinician over time (Varni, 1983).

Motivation

Adherence may be reinforced through verbal and written praise as well as tangible incentives (Friman, 2021a) such as token reinforcement (Varni, 1983), financial incentives (Shriver & Allen, 2008), or through collaborative development of a self-reinforcement program (Levensky & O'Donohue, 2006). Care must be taken to ensure adherent behavior is reinforced so as to outcompete existing reinforcers for nonadherent behavior (Moore & Amado, 2021). Predictability can protect against nonadherence, so discussion about benefits of adherence and the costs of nonadherence (Levensky & O'Donohue, 2006) and managing expectations regarding improvement (Watson, Foster, & Friman, 2006) can be helpful. Extinction bursts and social disapproval resulting from adherent behavior may be proactively established as signs of progress (Allen & Warzak, 2000).

Shriver and Allen (2008) recommend explaining that while child responsibility and independence are valuable goals, caregivers are an important part of the solution, and *everyone* will need to learn, and practice, new skills as part of successful treatment. Treatment may be sequenced to offer some immediate quick wins to give a sense of momentum (Allen & Warzak, 2000). Reviewing progress in graphical form, and noting how the data reflect adherence, can be highly motivating for caregivers. Making the entire learning process for the caregiver as fun and enjoyable as possible serves to improve adherence as well.

First Things First

Treatment outcomes can be sensitively dependent upon initial conditions. Caregivers struggling with marital challenges, sleep or other health problems, depression, anxiety, disorganization, substance overuse, or food or housing insecurity should be referred for treatment and help with accessing needed resources (Levensky & O'Donohue, 2006; Shriver & Allen, 2008). Prescriptive behavioral treatment could be offered in group format to serve as a support group for socially isolated caregivers (Shriver & Allen, 2008). In behavioral pediatrics, the treatment team includes the caregiver, and the caregiver, just like the clinician, must have sufficient resources to bring their A game. The family's readiness to begin treatment may be examined by asking caregivers about their concerns and beliefs about treatment, adherence with previous treatment, and confidence in their ability to implement recommendations (Levensky & O'Donohue, 2006). Problematic rule-governed management strategies (e.g., "You can't let some things go") will hopefully be identified and effectively addressed (Moore & Amado, 2021).

Caregiver Skill Acquisition

In behavioral pediatrics as in applied behavior analysis generally, the clinician assumes responsibility for outcomes and therefore assumes responsibility for caregiver adherence. Programming for treatment adherence is a form of programming for generalization and maintenance, given that caregivers receive the training in clinic with the clinician present, and then are expected to implement recommendations outside of it and in our absence. Stokes and Baer, in their classic 1977 paper on generalization, advised teaching many forms of the desired response so they are more likely to be naturally reinforced elsewhere, "training loosely" so that a wider range of stimuli evoke the trained response, using intermittent rather than fixed schedules of reinforcement, training in simulated conditions, incorporating self-reinforcement strategies, and reinforcing generalization itself as an operant.

How we teach is important to adherence rates and overall effectiveness (Allen & Warzak, 2000; Friman, 2021a), and anything we would want caregivers to do with their children we likely would want to model in training caregivers. Procedures for teaching new skills covered in Chapter 4, such as teach-back and behavioral skills training, may be applied by the practitioner when training caregivers. Miles and Wilder (2009), for example, demonstrated the effectiveness of using behavioral skills training to teach caregivers how to implement guided compliance procedures with their children.

Generally, simple language should be used (Levensky & O'Donohue, 2006; Moore & Amado, 2021; Shriver & Allen, 2008; Watson, Foster, & Friman, 2006) and the simpler the skill, the better adherence tends to be (Allen & Warzak, 2000). Procedures should be worded with high specificity (Cohrs et al., 2016; Levensky & O'Donohue, 2006) and may be in if-then format (Cohrs et al., 2016).

Procedures for caregiver implementation may be taught verbally as well as via modeling (Watson, Foster, & Friman, 2006), role play and behavioral rehearsal (Levensky & O'Donohue, 2006), and with visual aids (Levensky & O'Donohue, 2006; Shriver & Allen, 2008). Detailed instructions should be provided in writing (Levensky & O'Donohue, 2006; Watson, Foster, & Friman, 2006) and may be in the form of modular treatment protocols and handouts (discussed in Chapter 4) covering specific content for specific goals (discussed in Chapters 6 through 10). The environment in which caregiver training is offered should be free from distractions (Allen & Warzak, 2000; e.g., asking them to silence their phones while in session, and hiring a babysitter so no children are in the training room unless participating). Caregiver comprehension may be assessed via the teach-back procedure (see Chapter 4) or via observation (Levensky & O'Donohue, 2006). Performance feedback would then be offered (Cohrs *et al.*, 2016; Watson, Foster, & Friman, 2006).

Moore and Amado (2021) recommend relying not just on contingency-maintained adherent behavior, but on the development of rule governance as well. Helping caregivers develop self-management strategies is an option (Friman, 2021a), as is obtaining firm verbal commitments regarding specific treatment-related behaviors (Levensky & O'Donohue, 2006).

Facilitating Implementation

My typical practice mirrors that of Kazdin (2005): "Tasks are introduced, and trained gradually in the parent(s) ... based on the parent's execution of these tasks, the program continues, and new or varied tasks are introduced. If performance falters, if parent adherence is poor, or if the parent complains, the tasks can be reduced" (p. 192). Sometimes adherence may be improved by couching the prescribed procedures as an experiment (McNeil & Hembree-Kigin, 2010). Prompts should be incorporated in the treatment process to ensure families keep their appointments and implement recommended procedures as planned. Reminder calls have recently been replaced by automated email and text messages and are an effortless form of prompting for most practitioners. Adherence reminders may also come in the form of handouts and modular protocols, posted checklists, and the use of technology (e.g., prompting caregivers to set alerts on their phone for later self-prompting). Jones and her colleagues (2021) demonstrated how a homework checklist and daily text reminders to follow through and for appointments, along with daily surveys and video recording of skills practice and access to the clinician and skills videos for review and for showing family members, resulted in higher caregiver adherence and overall treatment efficiency with a course of behavioral parent training. Prompting via smart watch is also an option (e.g., White *et al.*, 2021).

Caregivers should be assisted in scheduling implementation around likely conflicts (Shriver & Allen, 2008) and taught to remove or reduce distractions, such as mobile device notifications and unannounced visitors, during times when procedures are to be implemented (Moore & Amado, 2021). Others in the home who may be (inadvertently or otherwise) sabotaging implementation may be invited into the therapy process, and if they refuse or are otherwise unavailable, the caregiver may be trained in assertiveness and boundary-setting skills (McNeil & Hembree-Kigin, 2010). Caregivers may also be trained in how to best communicate with the clinician (Levensky & O'Donohue, 2006), and skills, sequences, and performance criteria may be adjusted as needed (Shriver & Allen, 2008). Lastly, the clinician should often stress the critical importance of consistent follow-through and to avoid inadvertently reinforcing nonadherence (e.g., avoiding saying socially ordinary but clinically unhelpful things like, "Oh, it's okay," when learning of nonadherence; McNeil & Hembree-Kigin, 2010).

Key Takeaways from this Chapter

• Treatment adherence, or the extent to which caregivers follow through with prescribed procedures, is critical for treatment success, yet nonadherence rates range from 20% to 50%. Research, however, helps us to anticipate, prevent, and correct nonadherence.

• Careful initial assessment, rapport building, good listening skills, limited jargon use, facilitation of self-prompting, collaborative goal setting and treatment planning, and reinforcement of adherent behavior, among other efforts, can all improve treatment adherence and prevent nonadherence. Stokes and Baer's (1977) paper on generalization may serve as guidance as to the promotion of treatment adherence, given that adherence is a form of generalized responding.

References

Allen, K. D., Barone, V. J., & Kuhn, B. R. (1993). A behavioral prescription for promoting applied behavior analysis within pediatrics. *Journal of Applied Behavior Analysis, 26*, 493–502.

Allen, K. D., & Warzak, W. J. (2000). The problem of parental noncompliance in clinical behavior analysis: Effective treatment is not enough. *Journal of Applied Behavior Analysis, 33*, 373–391.

Baer, D. M., Wolf, M. M., & Risley, T. R. (1987). Some still-current dimensions of applied behavior analysis. *Journal of Applied Behavior Analysis, 20*, 313–327.

Bailey, J. S. (1991). Marketing behavior analysis requires different talk. *Journal of Applied Behavior Analysis, 24*, 445–448.

Bailey, J., & Burch, M. (2010). *25 essential skills & strategies for the professional behavior analyst: Expert tips for maximizing consulting effectiveness.* Routledge.

Becirevic, A., Critchfield, T. S., & Reed, D. D. (2016). On the social acceptability of behavior-analytic terms: Crowdsourced comparisons of lay and technical language. *The Behavior Analyst, 39,* 305–317.

Chacko, A., Anderson, L., Wymbs, B. T., & Wymbs, F. A. (2013). Parent-endorsed reasons for not completing homework in group-based behavioral parent training for high risk families of youth with ADHD. *Behaviour Change, 30,* 262–272.

Chacko, A., Wymbs, B. T., Arnold, F. W., Pelham, W. E., Swanger-Gagne, M., Girio, E. L., & O'Connor, B. (2009). Enhancing traditional behavioral parent training for single mothers of children with ADHD. *Journal of Clinical Child and Adolescent Psychology, 38,* 206–218.

Chadwell, M. R., Sikorski, J. D., Roberts, H., & Allen, K. D. (2019). Process versus content in delivering ABA services: Does process matter when you have content that works? *Behavior Analysis: Research and Practice, 19,* 14–22.

Cohrs, C. M., Shriver, M. D., Burke, R. V., & Allen, K. D. (2016). Evaluation of increasing antecedent specificity in goal statements on adherence to positive behavior-management strategies. *Journal of Applied Behavior Analysis, 49,* 768–779.

Critchfield, T. S., Doepke, K. J., Epting, L. K., Becirevic, A., Reed, D. D., Fienup, D. M., Kremsreiter, J. L., & Ecott, C. L. (2017). Normative emotional responses to behavior analysis jargon or how not to use words to win friends and influence people. *Behavior Analysis in Practice, 10,* 97–106.

DiMatteo, M. R. (2004). Variations in patients' adherence to medical recommendations: A quantitative review of 50 years of research. *Medical Care, 42,* 200–209.

Fisher, W. W., Greer, B. D., Shahan, T. A., & Norris, H. M. (2023). Basic and applied research on extinction bursts. *Journal of Applied Behavior Analysis, 56,* 4–28.

Foxx, R. M. (1996). Translating the covenant: The behavior analyst as ambassador and translator. *The Behavior Analyst, 19,* 146–161.

Friman, P. C. (2014). Behavior analysts to the front! A 15-step tutorial on public speaking. *The Behavior Analyst, 37,* 109–118.

Friman, P. C. (2017). You are in the way! Opening lines of transmission for Skinner's view of behavior. *The Behavior Analyst, 40,* 173–177.

Friman, P. C. (2021a). Behavioral pediatrics: Integrating applied behavior analysis with pediatric medicine. In W. W. Fisher, C. C. Piazza, & H. S. Roane (Eds.), *Handbook of Applied Behavior Analysis* (2nd ed., pp. 408–426). Guilford.

Friman, P. C. (2021b). There is no such thing as a bad boy: The circumstances view of problem behavior. *Journal of Applied Behavior Analysis, 54,* 636–653.

Hineline, P. N. (1980). The language of behavior analysis: Its community, its functions, and its limitations. *Behaviorism, 8,* 67–86.

Jones, D. J., Loiselle, R., Zachary, C., Georgeson, A. R., Highlander, A., Turner, P., Youngstrom, J. K., Khavjou, O., Anton, M. T., Gonzalez, M., Bresland, N. L., & Forehand, R. (2021). Optimizing engagement in behavioral parent training: Progress toward a technology-enhanced treatment model. *Behavior Therapy, 52,* 508–521.

Kazdin, A. E. (1996). Dropping out of child therapy: Issues for research and implications for clinical practice. *Clinical Child Psychology and Psychiatry, 1,* 133–156.

Kazdin, A. E. (2005). *Parent management training: Treatment for oppositional, aggressive, and antisocial behavior in children and adolescents.* Oxford.

Lattal, K. A., & Neef, N. A. (1996). Recent reinforcement-schedule research and applied behavior analysis. *Journal of Applied Behavior Analysis, 29*, 213–230.

Levensky, E. R., & O'Donohue, W. T. (2006). Patient adherence and nonadherence to treatments. In W. T. O'Donohue & E. R. Levensky (Eds.), *Promoting treatment adherence: A practical handbook for health care providers* (pp. 3–14). Sage.

Lindsley, O. R. (1991). From technical jargon to plain English for application. *The Behavior Analyst, 24*, 445–448.

Maatar, M. E., & Yaffe, S. J. (1974). Compliance of pediatric patients with therapeutic regimens. *Postgraduate Medicine, 56*, 181–188.

McNeil, C. B., & Hembree-Kigin, T. L. (2010). *Parent-child interaction therapy* (2nd ed.). Springer.

Miles, N. I., & Wilder, D. A. (2009). The effects of behavioral skills training on caregiver implementation of guided compliance. *Journal of Applied Behavior Analysis, 42*, 405–410.

Moore, T. R., & Amado, R. S. (2021). A Conceptual Model of Treatment Adherence in a Behavior Analytic Framework. *Education and Treatment of Children, 44*, 1–17.

Moore, T. R., & Simons, F. J. (2011). Adherence to treatment in a behavioral intervention curriculum for parents with children with autism spectrum disorder. *Behavior Modification, 35*, 570–594.

Nock, M. K., & Kazdin, A. E. (2005). Randomized control trial of a brief intervention for increasing participation in parent management training. *Journal of Consulting and Clinical Psychology, 73*, 872–879.

Normand, M. P., & Donohue, H. E. (2022). Behavior analytic jargon does not seem to influence treatment acceptability ratings. *Journal of Applied Behavior Analysis, 55*, 1294–1305.

Patterson, G. R. (1976). The aggressive child: Victim and architect of a coercive system. In E. J. Mash, L. A. Hamerlynck, & L. C. Handy (Eds.), *Behavior modification and families* (pp. 267–316). Brunner/Mazel.

Rapoff, M. A. (2010). *Adherence to pediatric medical regimens* (2nd ed.). Springer.

Rogers, C. R. (1957). The necessary and sufficient conditions of therapeutic personality change. *Journal of Consulting Psychology, 21*, 95–103.

Rohrer, J. L., Marshall, K. B., Suzio, C., & Weiss, M. J. (2021). Soft skills: The case for compassionate approaches or how behavior analysis keeps finding its heart. *Behavior Analysis in Practice, 14*, 1135–1143.

Rolider, A., & Axelrod, S. (2005). The effects of "behavior-speak" on public attitudes toward behavioral interventions: A cross-cultural argument for using conversational language to describe behavioral interventions to the general public. In W. L. Heward, T. E. Heron, N. A. Neef, S. M. Peterson, D. M. Sainato, G. Cartledge, R. Gardner III, L. D. Peterson, S. B. Hersh, & J. C. Dardig (Eds.), *Focus on behavior analysis in education: Achievements, challenges, opportunities* (pp. 283–294). Pearson.

Sanders, M. R., & Glynn, T. (1981). Training parents in behavioral self-management: An analysis of generalization and maintenance. *Journal of Applied Behavior Analysis, 14*, 223–237.

Shriver, M. D., & Allen, K. D. (2008). *Working with parents of noncompliant children: A guide to evidence-based parent training for practitioners and students.* American Psychological Association.

St. Peter, C. C., Pence, S. T., & Kestner, K. M. (2017). Consultation practices: Multidisciplinary settings. In J. K. Luiselli (Ed.), *Applied behavior analysis advanced guidebook: A manual for professional practice* (pp. 285–305). Academic.

Stimson, G. V. (1974). Obeying doctor's orders: A view from the other side. *Social Science and Medicine, 8,* 97–104.

Stocco, C. S., & Thompson, R. H. (2015). Contingency analysis of caregiver behavior: Implications for parent training and future directions. *Journal of Applied Behavior Analysis, 48,* 417–435.

Stokes, T. F., & Baer, D. M. (1977). An implicit technology of generalization. *Journal of Applied Behavior Analysis, 10,* 349–367.

Target, M., & Fonagy, P. (2005). The psychological treatment of child and adolescent psychiatric disorders. In A. Roth & P. Fonagy (Eds.), *What works for whom? A critical review of psychotherapy research* (2nd ed.). Guilford.

Varni, J. W. (1983). *Clinical behavioral pediatrics: An interdisciplinary biobehavioral approach.* Pergamon.

Wahler, R. G. (1976). Deviant child behavior within the family: Developmental speculations and behavior change strategies. In H. Leitenberg (Ed.), *Handbook of behavior, modification, and behavior therapy* (pp. 516–543). Prentice Hall.

Watson, T. S., Foster, N., & Friman, P. C. (2006). Treatment adherence in children and adolescents. In W. T. O'Donohue & E. R. Levensky (Eds.), *Promoting treatment adherence: A practical handbook for health care providers* (pp. 343–351). Sage.

White, K. R., Radley, K. C., Olmi, D. J., & McKinley, L. E. (2021). Increasing teachers' use of behavior specific praise via Apple Watch prompting. *Psychology in the Schools.* 10.1002/pits.22622

Multidisciplinary Collaboration

12

Dr. Thomas Young was an Englishman who lived from 1773 to 1829; he is said to have been the last person to know just about everything there was to know (Robinson, 2005). He's the guy who proved Newton wrong as to the physics of light and, familiar with over 400 languages, successfully deciphered the Rosetta Stone. The march of science and the associated exponential increase in things to know since his time have unfortunately rendered a polymath of today no chance at Dr. Young's title, and has left us dependent upon each other in our efforts to solve problems of modern living. No one person can know everything anymore. We simply must collaborate.

This is particularly true when it comes to behavioral health. "The understanding and application of effective mental health treatment," wrote Greydanus and Wolraich (1992), "requires an interdisciplinary team of professionals – primary care professionals, psychologists, psychiatrists, family therapists, behavioral (developmental) pediatricians, and others. No one holds the golden key to comprehend and accomplish it all" (p. ix). The very first interdisciplinary collaboration by behavior analysts on record, in fact, was with nurses in the very first published demonstration of applied behavior-analytic treatment (i.e., Ayllon & Michael, 1959). Fast forward to today and you'll find the author regularly collaborating with pediatricians, pediatric gastroenterologists and urologists, pediatric neurologists, child and adolescent psychiatrists, occupational therapists, mental health therapists, clinical social workers, dietitians, and educators as well as fellow behavior analysts and even horseback riding and martial arts instructors. We support, learn from, and encourage each other, all to the advantage of our clients and their families.

DOI: 10.4324/9781003371281-13

Entering the orbit of professionals from other disciplines through collaboration has taught me quite a lot through the years. Less than a third of psychologists report feeling confident with respect to collaborating with medical professionals (American Psychological Association, 2016), yet pediatricians, for example, tend to be highly supportive of requests for ride-alongs during hospital rounds and office visits and are impressed when encountering interest in doing so. Besides boosting confidence, seeking to actively collaborate with multidisciplinary peers serves as a hedge against the *unknown unknown* – the dreaded "unk-unk" – of Donald Rumsfeld fame; that is, you don't know what you don't yet know that may be important in the care of your client and in collaboration with others. The reader is encouraged to seek out and take advantage of as many opportunities to learn from professionals of other disciplines as possible.

Our multidisciplinary colleagues are also susceptible to the unk-unk phenomenon. I have encountered superb pediatricians who were unaware that tics are not purely neurologic in origin and are often rapidly amenable to behavioral treatment, and intelligent, committed pediatric gastroenterologists whose go-to for encopresis was MiraLAX without real consideration of the role of behavioral factors. Pediatric neurologists and child and adolescent psychiatrists are often dazzled when first presented with continuous measurement data on mutual clients, offering them granular analyses of the effects of changes in prescribed medication and dosage and the relative effects of behavioral treatment components. Such moments make the behavior analyst smile during the drive home from work. The science of behavior analysis remains enigmatic to those not trained in it yet nearly everyone given an opportunity to apply the science to their own work or see it in action with their clients is left wondering where it has been their whole lives.

Multidisciplinary collaboration also allows the rule-out, or identification and treatment, of medical conditions prior to the implementation of behavioral treatment. I now routinely require an ophthalmological examination prior to the behavioral treatment of acute onset eye tics given that a percentage of cases within the practice have been found to be secondary to corneal abrasion; in such cases, it is the abrasion that needs addressing, not the eye blinking. I have also learned to work in concert with pediatricians and pediatric endocrinologists in cases of sudden onset depression in teens especially when there is family history of hypothyroidism; in such cases, it may be Hashimoto's disease causing what appears to client and family (and psychiatrist!) to be depression. And taking a page from Pace and Toyer (2000), mouthing and pica are always first assumed to be secondary to a nutritional deficiency. The ability to solve "oral fixations" with just a multivitamin can be dumbfounding for parents and multidisciplinary colleagues alike.

Such scenarios – eye tics caused by corneal abrasions, depression caused by low thyroxine, and mouthing caused by nutritional deficiency – involve what are known colloquially as *masquerading conditions*, medical or biological conditions that topographically present as behavioral health concerns (Schildkrout, 2011; Taylor, 2007). Rates of misdiagnosis along these lines are not established for the pediatric population but among adults receiving behavioral healthcare services the rates are estimated to reach 19% (Taylor, 2007). It stands to reason that nonmedical behavioral health practitioners are much less likely than physicians to identify masquerading conditions (Grace & Christensen, 2007) as most behavioral health providers are not medically trained. But we can do better, and remaining current with the literature (see, for example, Copeland & Buch, 2020) and actively collaborating with and learning from our physician colleagues serve to improve healthcare for everyone. Such is ethical practice; the Ethics Code for Behavior Analysts requires that behavior analysts "collaborate with colleagues from their own and other professions in the best interest of clients and stakeholders" (Standard 2.10), "ensure, to the best of their ability, that medical needs are assessed and addressed if there is any reasonable likelihood that a referred behavior is influenced by medical or biological variables" (Standard 2.12), and "arrange for appropriate consultation with and referrals to other providers in the best interests of their clients" (Standard 3.06).

Relatedly, the unintended effects of prescribed medications should be considered; psychostimulant use, for example, often suppresses appetite which alters the reinforcing nature of food (Newhouse-Oisten *et al.*, 2017). This would be a critical consideration in the treatment of picky eating, and collaboration with the prescribing physician can make a big difference for the client and family.

Models of Professional Collaboration

Professional collaboration may be conceptualized along multidimensional continua from *multidisciplinary* to *interdisciplinary* to *transdisciplinary* along one dimension (e.g., Interprofessional Education Collaborative, 2016), and *coordinated* to *colocated* to *integrated* services along another dimension (e.g., National Council for Mental Wellbeing, 2020). The first dimension reflects the extent of active collaboration whereas the second reflects the extent of proximity. Professionals from different disciplines may collaborate in client care to a little or large extent and they may be housed or not housed in the same location or employed by each other.

With this multidimensional model in mind, multidisciplinary collaboration is relatively siloed as to decision making and represents a simple sharing of information, whereas interdisciplinary collaboration represents more of a team approach to decision making. Transdisciplinary collaboration, alternatively, is characterized by a liberalization of professional roles and is typically found in arena assessment situations, such as early intervention assessment conducted simultaneously by a psychologist and speech, physical, and occupational therapists (Slim & Reuter-Yuill, 2021). This model, however, appears susceptible to ethical problems, given blurred lines as to the scope of practice (LaFrance et al., 2019; see also, for example, the Ethics Code for Behavior Analysts Standards 1.04 Practicing within a Defined Role, 1.05 Practicing within Scope of Competence, and 2.01 Providing Effective Treatment) and requires strong teamwork to function. Of the three models along this first dimension, the interdisciplinary model, generally speaking, appears the most viable (Englander et al., 2013).

As for the second dimension of this multidimensional model comprised of coordinated, colocated, and integrated services, coordinated services are characterized by relatively minimal professional collaboration with sparse communication at a distance, colocated services refer to the same location and therefore more access and contact, and integrated services refer to close, consistent teamwork. Service delivery, patient experience, and organizational commitment and business model vary greatly across this dimension with each level of collaboration having its own advantages and disadvantages. On the one hand, independent decision making in private practice (i.e., coordinated services) is very nice, but on the other hand, multidisciplinary communication is made much easier within integrated settings under an interdisciplinary or transdisciplinary model and many clients may benefit much more from such a team-based approach.

Colocation refers to behavioral healthcare providers locating their services under the same roof as primary care physicians. They remain separate legal entities, however, while the waiting room, scheduling and reception services, and break room may be shared. This arrangement offers the behavioral healthcare provider relatively more autonomy than integration. I have maintained colocation arrangements with pediatric practices in the past, and found it highly advantageous for all parties. Such an arrangement offers mutual benefits in terms of referrals, increased familiarity among the represented disciplines, and ease of communication among the providers. Also, stigma surrounding behavioral health services is reduced when such services are housed within a medical facility (Gatchel & Oordt, 2003).

Full integration, on the other hand, refers to behavioral healthcare providers serving under the legal entity of the medical practice in which they are colocated, with a much greater degree of interdisciplinary collaboration per case. This model at its best offers the primary care patient truly comprehensive, superior care. Most children referred for behavioral health services under this arrangement actually receive them; Stancin and Perrin (2014) reported that whereas only 4% to 17% of children receive outside behavioral health services to which they were referred, closer to 95% accessed recommended services housed within the primary care setting. This phenomenal difference appears to be from more than just warm handoffs, or personal introductions of clients made by physicians (Pace et al., 2018). Full integration allows the behavioral healthcare provider to offer screenings and single-session contacts with families during which prescriptive behavioral treatment and health education may be offered (see Chapter 4), all during the same appointment made with the physician. Whereas behind-the-scenes hallway consultations between behavioral healthcare providers and physicians occur under the *colocation* model, such collaboration may be more formal and systematically planned under the *integrated* model.

Gatchel and Oordt (2003) discuss two other options: those of behavioral health consultant to primary care physicians (or what may be called the *brief consultation approach*), and staff adviser. In their view, the consultant acts as a care navigator following case review with physicians, sees their patients with behavioral health needs for one or two sessions, makes recommendations to primary care case managers and other physicians, monitors progress, and acts as a conduit between families and physicians. The consultant also offers presentations for groups of families whose children are high utilizers of medical care. This option falls along the continua closer to the interdisciplinary and integrated models. The option of staff adviser, on the other hand, does not involve seeing patients but simply serving as an expert consultant to the physicians who reach out for consultation on certain cases. This is likely not all a behavioral healthcare provider in this role would do with their day; the behavior analyst with expertise in behavioral pediatrics might see his or her own clients and serve as adviser to a number of primary care physicians or practices. Thus, the staff adviser model of collaboration would qualify as a coordinated but not necessarily colocated arrangement.

Competencies for Interdisciplinary Collaboration

Slim and Reuter-Yuill (2021) propose that the field of behavior analysis consider the Interprofessional Education Collaborative's (IPEC, 2016) competences for interdisciplinary collaboration and join organizations such as the American Psychological Association, American Council of Academic Physical Therapy, American Occupational Therapy Association, Association of Schools of Allied Health Professions, and Council on Social Work Education, and others who have taken the additional step of becoming recognized as institutional members or supporting organizations. Its four core competences and examples of listed sub-competences are offered below as a guide for practice.

- *Values/Ethics for Interprofessional Practice.* Work with individuals of other professions to maintain a climate of mutual respect and shared values.
  - Place interests of patients and populations at the center of interprofessional health care delivery and population health programs and policies, with the goal of promoting health and health equity across the lifespan.
  - Develop a trusting relationship with patients, families, and other team members.
  - Manage ethical dilemmas specific to interprofessional patient/population-centered care situations.
- *Roles/Responsibilities.* Use the knowledge of one's own role and those of other professions to appropriately assess and address the health care needs of patients and to promote and advance the health of populations.
  - Communicate one's roles and responsibilities clearly to patients, families, community members, and other professionals.
  - Engage diverse professionals who complement one's own professional expertise, as well as associated resources, to develop strategies to meet specific health and health care needs of patients and populations.
  - Forge interdependent relationships with other professions within and outside of the health system to improve care in advance learning.
- *Interprofessional Communication.* Communicate with patients, families, communities, and professionals in health and other fields in a responsive and responsible manner that supports a team approach to the promotion and maintenance of health and the prevention and treatment of disease.

- Communicate information with patients, families, community members, and health team members in a form that is understandable, avoiding discipline-specific terminology when possible.
- Express one's knowledge and opinions to team members involved in patient care and population health improvement with confidence, clarity, and respect, working to ensure a common understanding of information, treatment, care decisions, and population health programs and policies.
- Give timely, sensitive, instructive feedback to others about their performance on the team, responding respectfully as a team member to feedback from others.

- *Teams and Teamwork.* Apply relationship-building values and the principles of team dynamics to perform effectively in different team roles to plan, deliver, and evaluate patient/population-centered care and population health programs and policies that are safe, timely, efficient, effective, and equitable.
  - Integrate the knowledge and experience of health and other professions to inform health and care decisions, while respecting patient and community values and priorities/preferences for care.
  - Engage self and others to constructively manage disagreements about values, roles, goals, and actions that arise among health and other professionals and with patients, families, and community members.
  - Use process improvement to increase the effectiveness of interprofessional teamwork and team-based services, programs, and policies.

Supporting these goals are recent papers by, for example, LaFrance and colleagues (2019), who offer informative background on psychology, speech-language pathology, and occupational therapy, and Boivin and colleagues (2021), who share their training model and offer a helpful annotated bibliography. Allen, Barone, and Kuhn's (1993) paper offers great advice on how to become a valued collaborator with physicians, as does Newhouse-Oisten and colleagues' (2017) paper, which focuses on medication (see also Li & Poling, 2018, for helpful data from the field).

Bailey and Burch's (2023) *25 Essential Skills* represents a veritable finishing school for behavior analysts, considering what makes interdisciplinary collaboration successful and effective. It touches upon professional etiquette, professional leadership, managing challenges, networking, dealing with stress, public speaking, and critical thinking. Some wonderful advice on presentation skills is provided by Friman (2014, 2017), including using clear language, managing your own anxiety, commanding the audience's attention, intentionally and effectively using nonverbal behavior (e.g., posture and vocal volume, tempo, and tone), and maintaining topical relevance, among other considerations. Chapter 6 of this book offers lots of information on sleep health which will allow more effective collaboration with sleep specialists.

Barriers to Effective Collaboration

Barriers exist to multidisciplinary collaboration and should be anticipated. One particularly common barrier to effective collaboration between behavior analysts and professionals of other disciplines pertains to standard of care. Behavior analysts are held to the standard of science-based practice (e.g., Ethics Code for Behavior Analysts Standard 3.12 Advocating for Appropriate Services), and are expected to actively work to reduce or eliminate barriers to their treatment delivery and effectiveness (Standard 2.19 Addressing Conditions Interfering with Service Delivery). What should a behavior analyst do when encountering a multidisciplinary colleague who is doing scientifically questionable assessment or treatment with the behavior analyst's client?

Based on the Ethics Code and the current literature (e.g., Brodhead, 2015; LaFrance *et al.*, 2019; Miliotis & Weiss, 2021; Newhouse-Oisten *et al.*, 2017; Walmsley & Baker, 2019), behavior analysts should engage in effective consultation skills, ask questions and familiarize themselves with the treatment in question, make known their commitment to the Code, advocate for client safety, suggest that the treatment of concern be measured as to effectiveness *for this particular client* using a single-subject experimental design, and advocate for continued use of treatments or treatment components having demonstrable effectiveness and discontinuation of treatments or treatment components failing to show effectiveness. Additionally, Brodhead (2015) offers a checklist for use by behavior analysts, covering considerations such as whether a particular treatment is function-based and continuous measurement is planned, results in skill acquisition and promotes social competence and inclusion, has acceptable social validity and programs for sufficient treatment fidelity and adherence, and is within the logistical means of the family. An alternative guide for navigating such waters was put forth by Newhouse-Oisten and colleagues (2017).

Such a scenario is discussed by Gasiewski and colleagues (2021) involving collaboration between behavior analysts and pediatric occupational therapists. Behavior analysts practicing behavioral pediatrics will inevitably serve children who are also being served by occupational therapists offering sensory integration therapy, an approach widely considered pseudoscientific (American Academy of Pediatrics, 2012; Capuano & Killu, 2021; Freeman, 2007; Smith, Mruzek, & Mozingo; 2005; National Autism Center; 2009, 2015) and demonstrably inferior to behavior-analytic conceptualization and treatment (Mason & Iwata, 1990). While the soundness and selection of such sensory-based approaches may be questionable, it would be an error to conflate sensory approaches with occupational therapy generally. As Gasiewski and colleagues appropriately note, occupational therapists do far more for children than apply sensory therapies; they work to improve fine motor skills, teach calming skills, evaluate the need for and select adaptive equipment, and like behavior analysts, task analyze activities of daily living and develop treatment plans with consideration of among other factors the child's fine motor skills and physical environment. In other words, behavior analysts and occupational therapists have much more in common than they do not, and the skill sets of each are largely complementary. Behavior analysts will appreciate the occupational therapy field's very recent move toward evidence-based practice (American Occupational Therapy Association, 2020) and recent calls from within the field of occupational therapy to actively collaborate with behavior analysts (Scheibel & Watling, 2016; Whiting & Muirhead, 2019) and to even adopt behavior-analytic approaches (Welch & Polatajko, 2016). The Whiting and Muirhead (2019) paper in particular should be required reading for behavior analysts who regularly collaborate with occupational therapists.

Gasiewski and colleagues (2021) also note that *eclectic intervention* – a hodge-podge of interventions, some empirically supported and some not, from different professionals for a particular client – is known to be inferior to intensive behavioral intervention for children with autism (e.g., Howard *et al.*, 2005; Howard *et al.*, 2014). A distinction however should be drawn between eclectic intervention and collaborative treatment when all treatment components are empirically supported (see also Odom *et al.*, 2012). The main point of collaboration, we should remember, is to improve client care; when professionals from multiple disciplines each bring their best work, collaboration can be superior to the contributions of only one professional.

The fundamental differences between the biomedical and behavior-analytic approaches to problem conceptualization discussed in detail in

Chapter 2 can also make multidisciplinary collaboration challenging. Such challenges may be prevented by accepting differences in worldviews during interdisciplinary consultations and meetings and saving the philosophical conversation for collegial after-hours networking. Discussion of the application of behavior analysis across diagnoses and even independent of the diagnostic system is an example. Behavior analysts with experience in the public schools will be familiar with the Response to Intervention (RtI) approach (Hughes & Dexter, 2011). Historically, the identification and classification of learning disability (the educational version of diagnosis) for a child who couldn't read came first and the remediation (the educational version of treatment) came second. The point of RtI, alternatively, has been to treat first, and classify second *if needed*. Psychiatry's version of this is called *stepped diagnosis* (Batstra *et al.*, 2014; Frances, 2013), involving offering the least-intensive likely helpful treatment while delaying diagnosis and gradually arriving at a more definitive case formulation based on response. The American Academy of Pediatrics' recommendation to refer to a course of behavioral parent training *prior to diagnosing ADHD* in young children (Wolraich *et al.*, 2019) is an example of this practice in general medicine. The larger point here is that diagnosis is not required for treatment within general and specialty medicine and discussing RtI with educators and stepped diagnosis with physicians offers clarity for them as to how we can do what we do extradiagnostically. Additionally, Bowman and Weiss (2022) note that traditional problem conceptualization and treatment recommendations of multidisciplinary colleagues may be translated into behavioral principles for ourselves, a process that can help us identify conceptually sound interventions. Such a process may serve to find more common ground between collaborators of different training backgrounds.

The bottom line is that behavior analysts who actively collaborate with their multidisciplinary peers will be more effective for their clients and enjoy a much more rewarding career. As Slim and Reuter-Yuill (2021) note, multidisciplinary collaboration has been of interest to those in medicine for decades now. Behavior analysts, representing a fledgling profession, may be late to the party. Time to join.

Key Takeaways from this Chapter

- Multidisciplinary collaboration, when all treatment recommendations and components are empirically supported, results in superior client care over the efforts of a single provider.

- Forms of professional collaboration may be viewed as ranging from multidisciplinary to interdisciplinary to transdisciplinary in terms of extent of collaboration per case, and from coordinated to colocated to integrated in terms of extent of proximity. Multidisciplinary collaboration represents simple information sharing, interdisciplinary collaboration represents more of a team approach to decision making, and transdisciplinary collaboration represents an integration of disciplines with blurred boundaries for each discipline. Coordinated services are characterized by relatively minimal professional contact, colocated services are housed together with relatively more collaboration, and integrated services represent close, consistent teamwork within the same legal entity. Each form involves tradeoffs.
- Competencies for professional collaboration were discussed, involving values and ethics, roles and responsibilities, communication, and teamwork. Becoming familiar with roles, responsibilities, and challenges experienced by professionals of other disciplines, continuously improving one's professionalism, and anticipating and overcoming barriers to effective collaboration increase the value a clinician brings to the table and make for improved outcomes for children and their families.

References

Allen, K. D., Barone, V. J., & Kuhn, B. R. (1993). A behavioral prescription for promoting applied behavior analysis within pediatrics. *Journal of Applied Behavior Analysis, 26,* 493–502.

American Academy of Pediatrics (2012). Policy statement: Sensory integration therapies for children with developmental and behavioral disorders. doi: 10.1542/peds.2012-0876

American Occupational Therapy Association (2020). Occupational therapy practice framework: Domain & process (4th ed.). *American Journal of Occupational Therapy, 74* (*Suppl. 2*), 1–87. doi: 10.5014/ajot.2020.74S2001

American Psychological Association (2016). *2015 APA survey of psychology health service providers.* Author.

Ayllon, T., & Michael, J. (1959). The psychiatric nurse as a behavioral engineer. *Journal of the Experimental Analysis of Behavior, 2,* 323–334.

Bailey, J., & Burch, M. (2023). *25 essential skills for the professional behavior analyst: From graduate school to chief executive officer* (2nd ed.). Routledge.

Batstra, L., Nieweg, E. H., Pijl, S., van Tol, D. G., & Hadders-Algra, M. (2014). Childhood ADHD: A stepped diagnosis approach. *Journal of Psychiatric Practice, 20,* 169–177.

Boivin, N., Ruane, J., Quigley, S. P., Harper, J., & Weiss, M. J. (2021). Interdisciplinary collaboration training: An example of a preservice training series. *Behavior Analysis in Practice, 14,* 1223–1236.

Bowman, K. S., & Weiss, M. J. (2022). Teaching graduate students to translate non-behavioral treatments into behavioral principles. *Behavior Analysis in Practice*, 10.1 007/s40617-022-00736-2

Brodhead, M. (2015). Maintaining professional relationships in an interdisciplinary setting: Strategies for navigating nonbehavioral treatment recommendations for individuals with autism. *Behavior Analysis in Practice*, 8, 70–78.

Capuano, A. M., & Killu, K. (2021). Understanding and addressing pseudoscientific practices in the treatment of neurodevelopmental disorders: Considerations for applied behavior analysis practitioners. *Behavioral Interventions*, 36, 242–260.

Copeland, L., & Buch, G. (2020). Addressing medical issues in behavior analytic treatment. *Behavior Analysis in Practice*, 13, 240–246.

Englander, R., Cameron, T., Ballard, A. J., Dodge, J., Bull, J., & Aschenbrener, C. A. (2013). Toward a common taxonomy of competency domains for the health professions and competencies for physicians. *Academic Medicine*, 88, 1088–1094.

Frances, A. (2013). *Saving normal: An insider's revolt against out-of-control psychiatric diagnosis, DSM-5, big pharma, and the medicalization of ordinary life*. William Morrow.

Freeman, S. K. (2007). *The complete guide to autism treatments: A parent's handbook: Make sure your child gets what works!* SKF.

Friman, P. C. (2014). Behavior analysts to the front! A 15-step tutorial on public speaking. *The Behavior Analyst*, 37, 109–118.

Friman, P. C. (2017). Practice dissemination: Public speaking. In J. K. Luiselli (Ed.), *Applied behavior analysis advanced guidebook: A manual for professional practice* (pp. 349–366. Academic.

Gasiewski, K., Weiss, M. J., Leaf, J. B., & Labowitz, J. (2021). Collaboration between behavior analysts and occupational therapists in autism service provision: Bridging the gap. *Behavior Analysis in Practice 14*, 1209–1222.

Gatchel, R. J., & Oordt, M. S. (2003). *Clinical health psychology and primary care: Practical advice and clinical guidance for successful collaboration*. American Psychological Association.

Grace, G. D., & Christensen, R. C. (2007). Recognizing psychologically masked illnesses: The need for collaborative relationships in mental health care. *Journal of Clinical Psychiatry*, 9, 433–436.

Greydanus, D. E., & Wolraich, M. L. (1992). *Behavioral pediatrics*. Springer-Verlag.

Howard, J. S., Sparkman, C. R., Cohen, H. G., Green, G., & Stanislaw, H. (2005). A comparison of intensive behavior analytic and eclectic treatments for young children with autism. *Research in Developmental Disabilities*, 26, 359–383.

Howard, J. S., Stanislaw, H., Green, G., Sparkman, C. R., & Cohen, H. G. (2014). Comparison of behavior analytic and eclectic early interventions for young children with autism after three years. *Research in Developmental Disabilities*, 35, 3326–3344.

Hughes, C. A., & Dexter, D. D. (2011). Response to intervention: A research-based summary. *Theory Into Practice*, 50, 4–11.

Interprofessional Education Collaborative (2016). *Core competencies for interprofessional collaborative practice: 2016 update*. Interprofessional Education Collaborative. https://ipec.memberclicks.net/assets/2016-Update.pdf

LaFrance, D. L., Weiss, M. J., Kazemi, E., Gerenser, J., & Dobres, J. (2019). Multidisciplinary teaming: Enhancing collaboration through increased understanding. *Behavior Analysis in Practice*, 12, 709–726.

Li, A., & Poling, A. (2018). Board Certified Behavior Analysts and psychotropic medications: Slipshod training, inconsistent involvement, and reason for hope. *Behavior Analysis in Practice, 11*, 350–357.

Mason, S. A., & Iwata, B. A. (1990). Artifactual effects of sensory-integrative therapy on self-injurious behavior. *Journal of Applied Behavior Analysis, 23*, 361–370.

Miliotis, A., & Weiss, M. J. (2021). Clinical corner: What are some ethical and practical considerations when collaborating with nonbehavioral service providers? *Association for Science in Autism Treatment, 18.* https://asatonline.org/research-treatment/clinical-corner/collaborating-with-nonbehavioral-service-providers/

National Autism Center (2009). *National standards project: Findings and conclusions.* National Autism Center.

National Autism Center (2015). *National standards project, phase 2: Findings and conclusions.* National Autism Center.

National Council for Mental Wellbeing (2020). Standard framework for levels of integrated care. www.thenationalcouncil.org/wp-content/uploads/2020/01/cihs_framework_final_charts.pdf

Newhouse-Oisten, M. K., Peck, K. M., Conway, A. A., & Frieder, J. E. (2017). Ethical considerations for interdisciplinary collaboration with prescribing professionals. *Behavior Analysis in Practice, 10*, 145–153.

Odom, S., Hume, K., Boyd, B., & Stabel, A. (2012). Moving beyond the intensive behavior treatment versus eclectic dichotomy: Evidence-based and individualized programs for learners with ASD. *Behavior Modification, 36*, 270–297.

Pace, C. A., Gergen-Barnett, K., Veidis, A., D'Afflitti, J., Worcester, J., Fernandez, P., & Lasser, K. E. (2018). Warm handoffs and attendance at initial integrated behavioral health appointments. *Annals of Family Medicine, 16*, 346–348.

Pace, G. M., & Toyer, E. A. (2000). The effects of a vitamin supplement on the pica of a child with severe mental retardation. *Journal of Applied Behavior Analysis, 33*, 619–622.

Robinson, A. (2005). *The last man who knew everything: Thomas Young, the anonymous polymath who proved Newton wrong, explained how we see, cured the sick, and deciphered the Rosetta Stone, among other feats of genius.* Pi.

Scheibel, G., & Watling, R. (2016). Collaborating with behavior analysts on the autism service delivery team. *OT Practice, 21*, 15–19.

Schildkrout, B. (2011). *Unmasking psychological symptoms: How therapists can learn to recognize the psychological presentation of medical disorders.* Wiley.

Slim, L., & Reuter-Yuill, L. M. (2021). A behavior-analytic perspective on interpersonal collaboration. *Behavior Analysis in Practice, 14*, 1238–1248.

Smith, T., Mruzek, D. W., & Mozingo, D. (2005). Sensory integrative therapy. In J. W. Jacobson, R. M. Foxx, & J. A. Mulick (Eds.), *Controversial therapies for developmental disabilities: Fad, fashion, and science in professional practice* (pp. 331–350). Lawrence Erlbaum.

Stancin, T., & Perrin, E. C. (2014). Psychologists and pediatricians: Opportunities for collaboration in primary care. *American Psychologist, 69*, 332–343.

Taylor, R. L. (2007). *Psychological masquerade: Distinguishing psychological from organic disorders* (3rd ed.). Springer.

Walmsley, C., & Baker, J. C. (2019). Tactics to evaluate the evidence based of a nonbehavioral intervention in an expanded consumer area. *Behavior Analysis in Practice, 12*, 677–687.

Welch, C. D., & Polatajko, H. J. (2016). Applied behavior analysis, autism, and occupational therapy: A search for understanding. *American Journal of Occupational Therapy, 70*, 7004360020p1-7004360020p5. doi: 10.5014/ajot.2016.018689

Whiting, C. C., & Muirhead, K. (2019). Interprofessional collaborative practice between occupational therapists and behavior analysts for children with autism. *Journal of Occupational Therapy, Schools, and Early Intervention, 12*, 466–475.

Wolraich, M. L., Hagan, J. F., Allan, C., Chan, E., Davison, D., Earls, M., Evans, S. W., Flinn, S. K., Froehlich, T., Frost, J., Holbrook, J. R., Lehmann, C. U., Lessen, H. R., Okechukwu, K., Pierce, K. L., Winner, J. D., Zurhellen, W., & Subcommittee on Children and Adolescents with Attention-Deficit/Hyperactivity Disorder (2019). Clinical practice guideline for the diagnosis, evaluation, and treatment of attention-deficit/hyperactivity disorder in children and adolescents. *Pediatrics, 144*, e20192528. doi: 10.1542/peds.2019-2528

Glossary

abbreviated HRT, simplified HRT An empirically-based, pared-down version of the original 13-component habit reversal training treatment package consisting of awareness training, incompatible replacement behavior, social support, and if needed, relaxation training

ABC continuous recording "ABC" refers to antecedent, behavior, and consequence, and recording can be of simple frequency count, partial interval, or momentary time sampling recording over a selected interval of time during which a problem behavior typically occurs

ABC narrative recording A less rigorous recording method involving recording antecedent conditions and apparent consequences whenever a target behavior occurs

absence seizures Seizures characterized by a blank stare lasting less than a minute but occurring up to 100 times a day; this nonconvulsive form of epilepsy is most common in childhood, tends to be outgrown, and often masquerades as the inattentive form of ADHD or day-dreaming

actigraphy Measurement approach involving the wearing of a watch-like device on the nondominant wrist to measure movement under the assumption that no movement likely represents sleep

adjunctive behavior "Time-filler" behaviors, the frequency of which increases as a side effect of other behaviors maintained by a reinforcement schedule

algorithm In the context of case formulation and treatment planning, a flowchart guiding decision making

alpha directives   Directives that are direct and authoritative in nature

amygdala   Bilateral brain regions implicated in the retention of emotionally charged experiences

analytic constructs   Intervening variables such as behavioral principles, e.g., positive reinforcement, which may be tested empirically

argumentum ab auctoritate   A fallacious argument that something is true because authorities say it is true

argumentum ad populum   A fallacious argument that something is true because most people think it is true

authoritative management   Parenting style characterized by warmth and encouragement, high expectations, firm and fair discipline, and proactive coaching instead of reactive correction

bedtime fading   Help for children not usually sleepy at bedtime, a new bedtime is set for 45 minutes before typical sleep onset, and bedtime is made earlier by 15 minutes each week until arriving at the desired bedtime

Bedtime Pass   Help for bedtime refusal and curtain calls, the child is offered a token at bedtime to be redeemed before onset of sleep for a minute of the caregiver's time to supportively handle an easily satisfied request; if not redeemed, it may be redeemed in the morning for a special treat or privilege

behavioral health consultant to primary care physicians   Also known as the brief consultation approach, in which the consultant acts as care navigator following case review with physicians, offers brief therapy, makes recommendations for other providers, monitors progress, facilitates communication between families and providers, and offers group presentations

behavioral momentum   The effect (and strategy) of attaining greater behavioral compliance with low-probability directives by first issuing a series of high-probability directives

behavioral noncompliance   The failure to initiate within ten seconds the follow-through of a directive issued by a caregiver or other legitimate authority figure

behavioral parent training   A science-based approach to treatment involving the training of caregivers in authoritative management practices such as differential attending, effective directive delivery, use of positive and negative consequences, and problem-solving

behavioral quietude   Lying still and quiet in a relaxed state while awaiting sleep onset

behavioral skills training   A teaching method involving the provision of verbal or written instructions, modeling of the skill for the learner, having the learner rehearse the new skill, and providing performance feedback

behavioral trap   Communities of reinforcement in the natural environment that potentially shape much more new behavior

beta directives   Directives that are indirect, like requests

biomedical model   A model holding problem behavior to be reflective of medical disease states caused by faulty genes, brain structure, or brain function

case formulation, case conceptualization   The bridge between initial assessment and treatment planning, representing a synthesis of all information, insights, and likely helpful treatment approaches and methods

central disorders of hypersomnolence   The name for severe daytime sleepiness despite sufficient overnight sleep, diagnosed as narcolepsy and idiopathic hypersomnia

chain schedules   Two or more sequentially presented simple schedules of reinforcement each with a correlated discriminative stimulus, with reinforcement delivery following the final link in the chain

chemical imbalance   An unproven hypothesis holding that problem behavior is caused by an imbalance of neurotransmitters in the brain

Child's Game   Counterpoint to the *Parent's Game*, the Child's Game refers to a brief daily free-play session during which the caregiver offers a high rate of noncontingent reinforcement that is withheld at the occurrence of problem behavior

circadian rhythm sleep-wake disorder   The name for the failure to maintain a regular sleep-wake cycle due to alterations of the circadian rhythm or misalignment between circadian rhythm and work or social schedule

circular logic   A fallacious argument involving reliance on the conclusion to validate the premise

cleanliness training   In the context of the treatment of enuresis, teaching a child how and requiring the child to perform all age-appropriate cleaning tasks associated with wetting

clinical behavior analysis   A specialty within applied behavior analysis dealing with the application of behavior analysis to the treatment of problem behavior traditionally characterized as mental disorders

clinical health psychology   A specialty area within psychology involving the provision of preventative and treatment services to primarily adults at the confluence of medical and mental health

clinical metafactor   Problem facets of clinical presentations that likely occasion and maintain other problem facets; the prioritized treatment of metafactors results in a snowball effect as goals are sequentially addressed

colocated A form of collaborative service delivery in which services are provided in the same location with more access to and contact with collaborating professionals

comprehensive behavioral intervention for tics A treatment package including simplified habit reversal training (awareness training, incompatible replacement behavior, social support, and relaxation training) plus inconvenience review, contingency management, and relapse prevention programming all with an eye to behavioral function

contingency analysis The examination of the relationship between environmental factors and behavior

contingency based delay In the context of toleration training, delivery of reinforcement is made contingent upon the child making a toleration response (e.g., saying "okay") as well as engagement in leisure items

contingency contracting Development of a written agreement between caregiver and child outlining expected behavior and reward to be earned

coordinated A form of collaborative service delivery characterized by relatively minimal professional collaboration with sparse communication at a distance

criterion-referenced testing Administration of a test usually of an academic nature to determine whether a specific standard has been met

curtain calls A colloquial term for when children leave the bedroom for bids for attention following goodnight

cusp Any behavior change that opens the door to other important behavior changes

daily behavior report card; school-home note A strategy involving daily performance ratings by the teacher shared with the caregiver who then delivers positive or negative consequences at home

delayed sleep phase A two-hour or more delay in sleep pattern

descriptive assessment One of three components of functional behavior assessment involving the use of interviews, questionnaires, and rating scales as well as direct observation of the target behavior within the context in which it usually occurs

developmental-behavioral pediatrics A specialty area within medicine representing primarily physicians' provision of medical services to children with behavioral health issues

diaphragmatic breathing Also called belly breathing, taking slow, deep breaths so that the lungs are filled to capacity

didactic training   Preprepared lessons largely verbally delivered by the clinician to the child or caregiver

differential attending   Offering positive reinforcement in the form of attention contingent upon desired behavior while placing problem behavior on extinction

eclectic intervention   A hodge-podge of concurrent interventions, perhaps some evidence-based and some not, from different professionals for a particular client

effective directive delivery   Issuing verbal directives in ways that reliably increase the probability of compliance, such as using physical proximity and single-step directives

enuresis   The name for urination anywhere other than the toilet that has no known medical cause for children 5 years of age and older

encopresis   The name for defecation anywhere other than the toilet for children 4 years of age and older

epigenetic   Referring to changes in cell function resulting from DNA methylation and histone acetylation among other mechanisms

errorless compliance training   A strategy involving the use of only high-probability directives for a time, allowing the child to find success with following directions and contact reinforcement, followed by the fading in of lower-probability directives

establishing operations   Motivational operation involving an environmental variable that increases the reinforcement value of a particular stimulus

exclusionary time-out   A variation of a behavioral intervention involving the withdrawal of reinforcement contingent upon problem behavior; *exclusionary* refers to physically moving the child away from the action

exposure, graduated exposure   In the context of treatment for anxiety, remaining in the presence of a feared or otherwise aversive stimulus; graduated exposure refers to gradually increasing proximity or intensity

extinction bursting   Refers to an initial increase in the rate of responding immediately following the discontinuation of reinforcement for a previously reinforced behavior

extradiagnostic   Referring to an approach to assessment and treatment without the need for traditional diagnostic categories in behavioral health

fixed schedules of reinforcement   Reinforcement is delivered after the target behavior has been exhibited a certain number of times

functional behavior assessment, functional analysis A systematic assessment of the relationship between environment and behavior, for the purposes of knowing what skills to teach and changes to make to the environment to influence behavior; functional analysis refers to the most comprehensive form of functional behavior assessment which involves the use of interviews, questionnaires, rating scales, direct observation, and systematic manipulation of environmental variables

functional communication training For problem behavior serving as mands, teaching appropriate replacement communicative behavior while placing the problem behavior on extinction

functionalism In the context of behavioral healthcare, a philosophy holding that behavior occurs not due to some internal cause but as a function of present and historical circumstances

fundamental attribution error A concept from social psychology; the general tendency to blame something neurological or characterological in others for their problem behavior or misfortunes while blaming circumstances for our own

gastroesophageal reflux When stomach acid enters and irritates the esophagus

generalization Term for the engagement of a new behavior or skill in situations other than the one in which the behavior or skill was learned

genotype The complete set of genetic material of an organism

Good Morning Light Help for early waking involving provision and training of a visual cue signaling approval for leaving the bed

grounding In the context of treatment for anxiety, referring to focusing attention on the present moment through the use of any number of strategies

habits Persistent and repetitive, largely mindless behaviors such as thumb sucking, hair pulling or twirling, and nail biting

habit covariance When habits co-occur, suggesting one may be indirectly treated by directly treating the other

Hirschsprung disease A rare birth defect involving inadequate innervation of the large intestine which impairs peristalsis

hyperthyroidism A medical condition in which the thyroid produces too much thyroxine

hypoglycemia A medical condition involving low blood sugar

hypothetical constructs Speculative concepts created to account for what is observed

hypoventilation Breathing that is too shallow to maintain sufficient oxygen level and to prevent increased concentration of carbon dioxide

idiographic   Characteristic of a functional, behavior-analytic view of behavior in which clients are evaluated as individuals with their own unique learning histories and present circumstances

impacted   In the context of bowel health and constipation, when stool cannot move through the large intestine

indirect assessment   Assessment employing a variable other than the target behavior that is thought to reflect it

individual differences   Characteristics that distinguish one individual from another that remain relatively stable over time and across situations

insomnia   The name for difficulty with sleep onset or maintenance

integrated   A form of collaborative service delivery in which collaborating professionals all serve under the legal entity of the medical practice in which they are colocated with a much greater degree of interdisciplinary collaboration per case

interdisciplinary   A form of professional collaboration characterized by more of a team approach to decision making

intermittent schedules of reinforcement   Reinforcement is delivered after the target behavior has been exhibited a variable number of times

intestinal motility   The movement and speed with which stool moves through the large intestine

in vivo training   The training of skills within the circumstances in which the skills are intended to be used

isolation time-out   A more restrictive variation of a behavioral intervention involving the withdrawal of reinforcement contingent upon problem behavior; *isolation* refers to physically moving the child to the bedroom or similar location

long-term potentiation   The strengthening of neural circuits resulting in what is colloquially called habit patterns or muscle memory

maintenance   Generalization across time

mand   A communicative operant that specifies a desired reinforcer

manualized disorder-specific treatment   Treatment that is procedurally standardized for a particular clinical diagnosis

masquerading medical concerns   Medical or biological conditions that topographically present as behavioral health concerns and lead to misdiagnosis and undertreatment

medical home   A healthcare service delivery model characterized by comprehensive, patient-centered, coordinated, accessible, and high-quality services

mentalism In the context of behavioral healthcare, a philosophy holding an assumption of an inner metaphysical dimension, such as the mind, that causes behavior

modified extinction, graduated extinction In the context of bedtime training, a treatment approach characterized by a relatively longer duration but emotionally more tolerable procedures for children and caregivers

modular treatment, modularity Referring to treatment components consisting of strategies and decision rules; shelf-ready standardized protocols

momentary time sampling An observational data collection method involving the recording of presence or absence of a target behavior at regular predetermined intervals, the result of which is expressed as percentage of intervals

motivating operations Variables which alter the value of specific reinforcers and thus have an effect on the probability of behavior

multidisciplinary A form of professional collaboration characterized by independent decision making and a simple sharing of information with those of other disciplines

multiple schedules Two or more randomly presented simple schedules of reinforcement each with a correlated discriminative stimulus, with reinforcement delivered according to the schedule in effect at the time of the target response

narcolepsy The name for recurrent excessive daytime sleepiness and bouts of sudden sleep onset during the day

negative reinforcement The strengthening of a behavior by its termination or avoidance of an aversive stimulus

negative reinforcement trap A short-term solution at long-term cost for caregivers when actively avoiding making the child uncomfortable thereby avoiding the experience of worsened behavior; relief for the caregiver reinforces caregiver avoidance

neurodivergent A description meaning atypical neurological development and functioning

neuroplasticity The process by which structural and functional changes in the brain occur in response to behavior and interaction with the environment

neurotypical A description meaning typical neurological development and functioning

night terrors A parasomnia occurring during non-REM sleep characterized by screaming and expression of intense fear

nocturnal seizures A form of epilepsy characterized by night waking, shouting or screaming, arm and leg movements, and confusion overnight

nomothetic Characteristic of a traditional behavioral health perspective of behavior in which clients are evaluated as to their relative position statistically within a reference group

non-exclusionary time-out A less restrictive variation of a behavioral intervention involving the withdrawal of reinforcement contingent upon problem behavior; *non-exclusionary* refers to the use of planned ignoring or removal of a specific reinforcing stimulus such as pausing a preferred video

non-fecal obstruction A blockage in the large intestine caused by malformation or intussusception of the intestine

norm-referenced testing Administration of a test that has been standardized on a group of individuals to determine relative standing statistically

obstructive sleep apnea A breathing disorder during sleep characterized by at least five halts in the breath cycle of more than ten seconds each

operant A behavior selected, shaped, and maintained by the context in which it occurs

parasomnias A category of phenomena involving behavior or experiences during sleep or sleep-wake transitions; these include night terrors, sleepwalking, sleep paralysis, and others

Parents' Game Counterpoint to the *Child's Game*, the Parent's Game refers to the remainder of the day during which the caregiver leads the child

pediatric psychology A specialty area within psychology involving the provision of services to children with medical conditions as well as behavioral concerns

periodic limb movement disorder Repetitive limb movements during sleep that disrupt sleep

peristalsis Involuntary muscle movements propelling food and by-product through the gastrointestinal tract

phenotype Gene expression, or observational characteristics, based upon genotype plus environmental influences

pivotal behavior Behavior change that results in collateral effects on future learning

placed on extinction Targeted for discontinuation of contingent reinforcement

positive reinforcement trap A short-term solution at long-term cost for caregivers when actively avoiding making the child uncomfortable; doing so results in positive interactions between child and caregiver, thereby reinforcing caregiver avoidance

Premack principle Making contingent the access to and engagement in a high-preference activity on the engagement of a low-preference behavior; thus, the high-preference activity functions as a reinforcer for the low-preference behavior

prescriptive behavioral treatment Behavioral treatment prescribed by the clinician for the caregiver to carry out in day-to-day life

primary care A clinical focus on prevention as well as amelioration of problems of low intensity that without treatment are predicted to worsen and ultimately require higher levels of care

primary care behavioral pediatrics A subspecialty within clinical behavior analysis, itself a specialty within applied behavior analysis, addressing the primary care behavioral healthcare needs of children via science-based assessment and treatment in collaboration with caregivers, pediatricians, and other pediatric healthcare providers

progressive muscle relaxation A stress management and relaxation technique involving the sequential tightening and releasing of muscle groups

projective testing Administration of a test involving client responses to relatively vague stimuli under the assumption that those responses meaningfully reveal useful unconscious content not otherwise obtainable

prone Lying belly down

reductionist From *reductionism*; a logical fallacy involving the oversimplification of the complex to the point at which important meaning and utility are lost

reifying From *reification*; a logical fallacy involving the regarding of an abstraction as concrete

reinforcement schedule thinning Gradually increasing the required interval or quality of responding for reinforcement

reinforcer identification, preference assessment A process by which potential reinforcers to be intentionally offered contingent upon desired behavior are identified

REM sleep A stage of sleep characterized by rapid eye movements, dream sleep, and much brain activity but general paralysis

response restriction In the context of tolerance training, removing the opportunity to mand at times when reinforcement for manding is unavailable

restless legs syndrome   Also known as Willis-Ekbom disease, a condition characterized by discomfort in the legs and the resulting need to move them to attain momentary relief

restricted operants   Behaviors evoked under highly specific conditions

retention control training   To increase bladder capacity, rewarding a child for postponing urination for increasingly longer intervals

scatterplot analysis   A method of data collection that helps uncover temporal patterns that may suggest functional relationships between environmental variables and behavior

scheduled awakening   In the context of treatment of nocturnal enuresis, awaking the child just before he or she typically wets and prompting a visit to the potty

secondary care   A clinical focus on cure (versus prevention or minimization of impairment from more chronic conditions)

self-quieting   A child's ability to self-calm when upset

serotonin hypothesis   One facet of the chemical imbalance theory, itself unproven

setting events   A general term referring to antecedent variables such as motivational operations

shaken baby syndrome   Brain injury from being shaken violently

staff adviser   A service delivery role involving provision of consultation to physicians

standard of care   The level of professional behavior at which the average prudent practitioner within a given professional community would practice given similar circumstances

stepped diagnosis   A process involving offering the least-intensive likely helpful treatment while delaying diagnosis and gradually arriving at a more definitive case formulation based on response

stage I sleep   A stage of sleep at the transition from wakefulness to sleep

stage II sleep   A stage of sleep characterized by light sleep

stage III sleep   A stage of sleep characterized by deep sleep and much less brain activity

Sleep Check   An intervention involving the caregiver promising a reward for being asleep when returning shortly after lights-out; this intervention essentially incentivizes pretending to be asleep, which allows the onset of behavioral quietude necessary for sleep onset

social skills instruction   Explicit training of task-analyzed behavioral steps that together comprise socially competent behavior for specific social situations

social validity Refers to the acceptability and perceived value of treatment

sudden infant death syndrome The unexplained death of an infant while sleeping

swaddling The practice of wrapping an infant comfortably and securely in a blanket

supine Lying face up

teach-back A teaching method involving verbally explaining specific procedural steps and requiring the trainee to teach back the information in his or her own words

temperament Biologically based individual differences such as sensitivity, adaptability, introversion/extroversion, and approach/avoidance

tertiary care A clinical focus on minimization of impairment from more chronic conditions (versus prevention or cure)

three-step guided compliance A compliance training procedure involving 1) issuing a verbal directive, 2) prompting from least to most intrusive for follow-through, and 3) moving to physical prompting for follow-through if needed

tics Sudden, repetitive motor movements or vocalizations

time-in Counterpoint to *time-out*, the provision of noncontingent social reinforcement in the absence of inappropriate behavior

time-out A behavioral intervention involving the withdrawal of reinforcement contingent upon problem behavior

token reinforcement A strategy involving the awarding of tokens contingent upon desired behavior to be later exchanged for rewards such as privileges or preferred items

topography The observable form of behavior

transdiagnostic Referring to an approach to assessment and treatment applicable across traditional diagnostic categories in behavioral health

transdisciplinary A form of professional collaboration characterized by close teamwork and even a blurring of professional roles

treatment adherence The extent to which caregivers follow through with prescribed procedures outside of the consultation session

treatment fidelity The extent to which the clinician delivers the treatment as designed

triage The process of sorting patients or conditions by urgency in the context of finite resources

type I polysomnography (PSG) A clinical sleep study, done in a sleep lab involving the assessment of brainwave activity via electroencephalography (EEG), eye movement activity via electrooculography

(EOG), muscle activity via electromyography (EMG), and cardiac activity via electrocardiography (EKG), as well as oxygen saturation, end-tidal carbon dioxide, and respiratory effort

unmodified extinction   In the context of bedtime training, a treatment approach characterized by saying goodnight and then, while monitoring to ensure safety, placing all bids for attention on extinction until morning

urine alarm   A treatment for nocturnal enuresis involving a sensor for moisture and an alarm alerting the child to the need to complete urination in the bathroom

videosomnography   Time-lapse video recording of sleep

Index

ABC (antecedent-behavior-consequence) continuous recording 53–54
absence seizures 72
acceptance and commitment therapy (ACT) 71
actigraphy 93–94
acute onset depression 83
adherence-associated behaviors 148
adjunctive behavior 138
age and sleep requirements 89
algorithm 2, 69
Allen, K. 4, 5, 106, 148, 163
Aloia, M. 89
Amado, R. S. 152
American Academy of Pediatrics (AAP) 4, 67–68
American Board of Professional Psychology (ABPP) 20–21
American Psychological Association 20
amygdala 33, 88, 129
analytic constructs 30
antidepressant medications 30
anxiety 127–129
applied behavior analysis (ABA) 5–6, 54, 57
argumentum ab auctoritate 31
argumentum ad populum 31
assessment: in behavioral pediatrics 49–58; of caregiver treatment adherence 147–148; clinical 46–49; of sleep health 89–94; in traditional behavioral healthcare 46–49

attention-deficit hyperactivity disorder (ADHD) 3, 19, 20, 31, 32, 35, 47, 68, 88–89, 93, 146, 166
authoritative management practices 67, 112

Baer, D. M. 36, 57, 151
Bailey, J. S. 2, 163
Balance Program 71
Barlow, D. H. 57–58
Barone, V. 4, 5, 163
bedtime fading 97
Bedtime Pass intervention 98
behavioral healthcare services 57
behavioral health consultant to primary care physicians 161
behavioral momentum 110
behavioral noncompliance: defined 105; treatment of 107–114; typical compliance rates 106
behavioral parent training (BPT) 67–68, 107
behavioral pediatrics: about 12–13; assessment in 49–58; pediatricians 14–16; practice 18, 55; related subspecialties 18–22; training pathways 16–18
Behavioral Pediatrics: Research and Practice (Russo & Varni) 18–19
behavioral quietude 92, 97
behavioral skills training (BST) 66, 110

behavioral topography 35, 138–139
behavioral trap 147
Behavior Analyst, The 6
Behavior Analyst Certification Board
    (BACB) 17, 19
behavior-analytic case formulation 80
behavior-analytic models 147
Bergner, R. M. 81
Bicard, D. F. 121
bidirectional causality 72
Binder, L. M. 121
biomedical model of mental illness 30–32
Blum, N. J. 22, 37–39
Board Certified Assistant Behavior Analyst
    (BCaBA) 17–18
Board Certified Behavior Analyst (BCBA)
    17–18
Board Certified Behavior Analyst –
    Doctoral (BCBA-D) 17–18
Bowman, L. G. 166
brief functional analysis 54–55
Brodhead, M. 164
Brumfeld, B. D. 106
Burch, M. 163

caregivers: basic teaching for 65–66;
    feedback for 69; impact of directives by
    38; interview 90–93; modular
    treatment for 68–69; and problems
    with treatment adherence 146–147;
    role in children's behavioral healthcare
    13–14; skill acquisition 151–152
    see also prescriptive behavioral
    treatment
caregiver treatment adherence:
    assessment of 147–148; facilitating
    implementation 152–153; overview
    145–147; programming for 148–151;
    skill acquisition 151–152
case formulation/case conceptualization:
    clinical metafactors 80–81; treatment
    planning 82–84
central disorders of hypersomnolence 94
chain schedules 120
chemical imbalance 30
Child Behavior Checklist and Conners
    Rating Scale 48
children of preschool age 121
Child's Game 109
Chorpita, B. F. 69
Christophersen, E. 4, 5, 97, 111

circadian rhythm sleep-wake disorder 94
circular logic 31
cleanliness training 132, 133
Clinical Behavioral Pediatrics: An
    Interdisciplinary Biobehavioral Approach
    (Varni) 18–19
clinical behavior analysis 12, 71
clinical health psychology, defined 20
clinical metafactors 69, 80–81, 105, 120,
    127, 132, 134, 136
cognitive behavioral therapy (CBT) 3
colic 129–131
colocation 160–161
Common, E. A. 57
communication, interprofessional 162–163
Compassionate Collaboration tool 164
compliance 51, 52, 65, 66, 70, 71, 83, 105,
    106–110, 120, 137, 145, 151
comprehensive behavioral intervention
    for tics (CBIT) 139
contingency analysis 13, 147
contingency-based delays 122–123
contingency contracting 107, 111
corporal punishment 39–40
COVID-19 pandemic and behavioral
    healthcare 15
Crabtree, V. 89
criterion-referenced testing 47
curtain calls 92, 95, 98
cusp 124

daily behavior report card 107, 108, 114
Daleiden, E. L. 69
Dawes, R. M. 3
daytime training of self-quieting skills
    96–97
delayed sleep phase 90, 94
delay intolerance 120–122
denial and delay, toleration of 121–122
descriptive assessment 53–55
developmental-behavioral pediatrics 18–20
diaphragmatic breathing 128
didactic training 69
differential attending 16, 67, 84, 108, 110,
    131, 136, 137, 138
direct behavioral assessment 93–94
Direct Instruction 33
directive delivery: and behavioral
    noncompliance 109; effective 109; and
    language development 38
Dixon, M. R. 121

doing *versus* saying 38–39
Donaldson, D. L. 113
DSM diagnosis 35–37, 82
DSM-5-TR 30
dyscalculia 33
dyslexia 33

eclectic intervention 165
Edwards, C. P. 106
effective directive delivery 38, 67, 107, 108, 109, 110, 111, 113, 135
encopresis 13, 39, 134–137
Endo, S. 121
enuresis 13, 132–134
epigenetic alterations 32–33, 36
errorless compliance training 107, 108, 109–110
Essential Skills (Bailey and Burch) 163
establishing operations 137
Ethics Code for Behavior Analysts 159, 160, 164
exclusionary time-out 108
exposure-based interventions 3, 15, 128–129
extinction bursting 120
extradiagnostic behavior analysis 36, 166

feedback: for caregivers 69; instructive 163
Ferber, R. 89
fixed schedules of reinforcement 151
fluoxetine (Prozac) 30–31
Forehand, R. L. 106
Friman, P. 4, 5, 6, 22, 37–39, 89, 111, 164
full integration 161
Full Scale IQ standard score 47
functional behavior assessment (FBA) 47–48, 52–55
functional brain abnormalities 32
functional communication response 125–126
functional communication training (FCT) 120
functionalism 40
function-based prevention 69–71
fundamental attribution error 31–32, 148

Gardner, H. 106
Gasiewski, K. 165
gastroesophageal reflux 130
Gatchel, R. J. 161
generalization of treatment 67, 71, 82, 84, 108, 151

genotype 33
Ghezzi, P. M. 121
Good Morning Light intervention 98
graduated exposure 128–129
graduated extinction 96
Gravina, N. E. 65
Green, C. M. 82, 122, 126
Greydanus, D. E. 157
grounding 128–129
guided compliance 66, 110

habits 95, 137–139
Hanf, C. 67
Hanley, G. P. 55, 70, 122
Hawkins, R. P. 82
Hayes, S. C. 34, 57–58
health education 94–95
Hirschsprung disease 135
Horner, R. H. 66
House-Tree-Person 48
hyperthyroidism 129
hypoglycemia 129
hypothetical constructs 30, 31, 36, 47, 48, 49
hypothyroidism 83
hypoventilation 92

idiographic assessment 46, 49
impacted child 135
impulsivity 121
incentivization system 136
indirect assessment 53
individual differences 37
insomnia 90, 94
integrated primary care settings 57, 159–161
interdisciplinary collaboration 160, 162–164
intermittent schedules of reinforcement 71, 151
interprofessional communication 162–163
Interprofessional Education Collaborative (IPEC) 162
intestinal motility 135
in vivo training 69
IQ testing 47
isolation time-out 113
Iwata, B. A. 53, 54, 55

Johnston, J. M. 82
Jones, D. J. 152
Jongsma, A. E. 82

Kazdin, A. E. 67, 152
Keilitz, I. 66
Klopack, E. T. 33
Kuhn, B. 4, 5, 89, 163

LaFrance, D. L. 163
Lane, K. L. 57
language development 38
Likert ratings 48, 58
long-term potentiation 32

maintenance 71, 82, 84, 108, 151
mands/manding 120, 122, 124–125
manualized disorder-specific treatment 68
masquerading medical concerns 159
McConahay, K. H. 97
medical adherence 16
medical nonadherence 145–146
meditation 33, 128–129
Meltzer, L. J. 89
mental illness, biomedical model of 30–31
mentalism 34–35
metafactors 80–81, 82, 83, 87, 105, 120, 124, 127, 132, 134, 135, 136
methylation 34
Miles, N. I. 151
Mindell, J. A. 89
MiraLAX 158
modified extinction approach 96
modularity 65, 68–69, 151
modular treatment 65, 68–69, 151
momentary time sampling 53, 93
Moore, T. R. 152
motivating operations 107
Muirhead, K. 165
multidisciplinary collaboration: barriers to 164–166; models of 159–161; overview 157–159
multiple schedules 120

narcolepsy 90
National Commission for Certifying Agencies 17
Ndoro, V. W. 66
needle phobia 15
Neef, N. A. 53–54, 121
negative reinforcement 54, 84, 107, 128, 137, 147, 149
Nelson, T. D. 57–58
neurodivergent children 11
neuroplasticity 32–34

neuropsychological test batteries 47
neuroscience and problem behavior 32–34
neurotypical children 11, 87, 106
New Age energy healing approaches 3
Newhouse-Oisten, M. K. 163, 165
night terrors 90, 92
nocturnal enuresis 132
nocturnal seizures 92
nomothetic assessment 46, 49
nonacceptance of decisions 120–122
non-exclusionary time-out 113
non-fecal obstruction 135
norm-referenced testing 47

objective measurement, assessment through 57–58
observation, assessment through 52
obstructive sleep apnea 90, 92
Oordt, M. S. 161
operant conditioning 33, 35, 55, 71, 92, 107, 134, 139, 147
oppositional defiant disorder 48
Owens, J. A. 89

Pace, G. M. 158–159
parasomnias 90, 92, 95, 133
parenting behavior 147
parent management training 67–68
Parent's Game 109
Patterson, G. R. 147
pediatricians 14–16
pediatric pain 15–16
pediatric psychology 20
Pennypacker, H. S. 82
periodic limb movement disorder 92
peristalsis 135
Perlis, M. 89
Perrin, E. C. 2, 161
Peterson, A. L. 53–54
phenotype 32–33
picky eating 83, 159
placed on extinction 122
Portillo, D. 65
positive reinforcement trap 147
practice locations 17–18
preference assessment 56, 57
Premack principle 112
premonitory sensations 137
preschool children 15, 22, 87, 89, 121, 125
Preschool Life Skills Program 70–71

preschool years, sleep problems during 87–88
prescriptive behavioral treatment: basic teaching for caregivers 65–66; behavioral parent training 67–68; function-based prevention 69–71; modular treatment for caregivers 68–69; overview 64–65 *see also* caregivers
preteens 125
primary care: behavioral pediatrics 11, 21–22, 46, 59, 64, 69; defined 12; medical providers 13–14, 72, 129, 132; settings 67 *see also* behavioral pediatrics
problem behavior conceptualization: alternative model 34–37; biomedical model of mental illness 30–32; critical considerations for 37–40; and neuroscience 32–34
progressive muscle relaxation 128–129
projection in mental measurement 48
projective testing 48
prone position 131
psychostimulants 159
punishment, impact of 39–40

questionnaires 50–51, 93

reductionism 31, 41
referral 72–73
Registered Behavior Technician (RBT) 17
reifying construct 31
reinforcement schedule thinning 120
reinforcer identification 56
REM sleep 90
repetition with contrast 39–40
response restriction 120
Response to Intervention (RtI) approach 166
restless legs syndrome (RLS) 90, 92
restricted operants 55
retention control training 132
Reuter-Yuill, L. M. 162, 166
reward programs 110–113, 126
Risley, T. R. 36
Roberts, M. W. 106
Rohrer, J. L. 164
Rorschach Inkblot Test 3, 48

scatterplot analysis 53
scheduled awakening 132, 133
school-age child 22, 125

school-home note 114
Schweitzer, J. B. 121
screener instruments 53
secondary care, defined 12
selective serotonin reuptake inhibitors (SSRIs) 30–31
self-advocacy skills 124–126
self-control 121
self-quieting 92, 96–97
serotonin hypothesis 31
setting events 107, 139
shaken baby syndrome 130
Shiffman, S. 52
Shriver, M. D. 106
Simons, F. J. 33
Skinner, B. F. 5, 35, 54, 57
sleep: diary 93; stages 90; terrors 95
Sleep Check 97–98
sleep habits 95
sleep health, assessment of: methods 90–94; sleep requirements by age 89; sleep stages 90
sleep-related problems, treatment of: bedtime fading 97; Bedtime Pass intervention 98; daytime training of self-quieting skills 96–97; flashlight treasure hunts 96; Good Morning Light intervention 98; health education 94–95; modified extinction approach 96; Sleep Check 97–98; unmodified extinction approach 95–96
Sleiman, A. A. 65
Slim, L. 162, 166
social skills instruction 71
social validity 50, 56–57, 58, 82, 164
staff adviser 161
Stancin, T. 2, 161
standard of care 164
Stanford marshmallow experiment 121
stepped diagnosis 166
Stocco, C. S. 147
Stokes, T. F. 151
Stone, A. A. 52
Strain, P. S. 106
structural brain abnormalities 32
structured interviews 53
sudden infant death syndrome 131
Sulzer-Azaroff, B. 121
supine position 131
supportive counseling 71–73
swaddling 131

teach-back method for caregivers 65
team dynamics and multidisciplinary
   collaboration 163
temperament and individual differences 37
tertiary care 12, 20, 29
Thompson, R. H. 147
three-step guided compliance 66, 71, 107, 110
thumbsucking 11
tics 137–139
Tierney, J. 122, 126
time-in intervention 109
time-out intervention 40, 110, 113
toileting problems 13, 135–137
token reinforcement 107, 114, 133, 150
toleration of denial and delay 121–122
topography, behavioral 35, 138–139
Toyer, E. A. 158–159
training pathways 16–18
transdiagnostic assessment 39, 68
transdisciplinary collaboration 160
treatment adherence see caregiver
   treatment adherence
treatment fidelity 3, 69, 145
triage 19
type I polysomnography (PSG) 92

unmodified extinction approach
   95–96
urges 137
urine alarm 132

videosomnography 93
visualization 128–129
Vlaeyen, J. W. S. 46
Vollmer, T. R. 113

Wahler, R. G. 147
Wallace, M. D. 55
Warzak, W. J. 148
Watson, T. S. 57
Wechsler Intelligence Scale for Children,
   Fifth Edition 47
Weiss, M. J. 166
Weisz, J. R. 69
Whiting, B. B. 106, 165
Wilder, D. A. 151
Wolf, M. M. 36, 56, 57
Wolraich, M. L. 157
Woodcock-Johnson achievement tests 47
Woodworth, R. 30–31

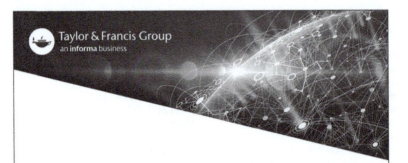

Printed and bound by CPI Group (UK) Ltd, Croydon, CR0 4YY
08/06/2025
01897008-0001